Don't go There ALONE!

A Guide to Hospitals for Patients and Their Advocates

Kathy Kalina, RN, CHPN

Stephen Pew, Ph.D.

Diane Bourgeois, LMSW

Published by 33-44-55 Publishing
6324 N. Chatham Avenue
Kansas City, MO   64151
E-mail: Publisher334455@aol.com
www.thepatientadvocate.org

ISBN: 0-9755549-0-5
Library of Congress Control Number 2004093984
Printed in the United States of America

This publication is designed to provide information and guidance with regard to the subject matter covered. It is sold with the understanding that the publisher and authors are not engaged in rendering legal, medical, accounting or other professional advice. If legal, medical or other expert assistance is required, the services of a competent, licensed professional person should be sought.

Adapted from a *Declaration of Principles* jointly adopted by a committee of the American Bar Association and a committee of publishers and associations.

Edited by:
J. Kathy Walker
Walker Texas Writer
Fort Worth, Texas

Cover Design:
Jennifer Henderson
Illustrations:
Barry Rodges
jodesign
Fort Worth, Texas

Dedication

This book is dedicated to those individuals who have served as health care advocates for a friend, a family member, a co-worker or even a stranger. Your courage and the stories you shared with us were essential to the development of this book. You have demonstrated the remarkable tenacity of the human spirit to care for others. Your seemingly inexhaustible strength and fierce determination to advocate for those who cannot advocate for themselves has humbled us. Just by your way of being you have taught us that no one need ever be alone. For these gifts, we shall always be grateful.

Table of Contents

Introduction

Imagine that you're going on the trip of a lifetime. From the very beginning you know there will be difficulties and inconveniences. You will spend time waiting for planes, trains and automobiles. Sometimes you'll be hungry or thirsty. There will be some communication problems and an absence of the comforts of home. You can expect a great deal of uncertainty and at least the possibility of danger, requiring a heightened level of vigilance. Through it all, a dog-eared copy of your travel guide will be your constant companion.

Travel guides spell out the local customs and idiosyncrasies of foreign cultures, and travelers depend on them for a reason: ignoring the "rules of the road" will bring inevitable consequences. These guides tell you when local customs might conflict with closely held values or personal safety, and instruct you to employ an experienced personal guide when you need help navigating dangers. Being prepared increases your chances of arriving at your destination safe and sound, prepared for the peak experience that eclipses all the mental strain, physical deprivation and financial sacrifice.

Our desire for good health is a similar journey. No one wakes up in the morning and says, "I'd really like to go to the hospital. I'm in the mood for a medical procedure. Maybe even a little surgery." We access the health care system to recover or improve our health, or to get relief from bothersome symptoms. Achieving the best possible quality of life is our ultimate goal. The hospital is a means to an end, not the destination. We are just passing through. This book is a travel guide to help the consumer arrive safe and sound on the other side of hospitalization.

The American hospital is a foreign culture with unspoken rules and mysterious customs. And the word is out that it's a very dangerous place to be. Every day in every hospital, patients get the wrong procedures, tests and medicines. Communication gets garbled. Requests get ignored. Mistakes happen. Hospital acquired infections and errors cause an untold amount of misery. Because of chronic under-reporting, we have no idea how many patients suffer complications, delayed recovery and permanent injury. There are estimates of 30,000 to 60,000 deaths per year from medical errors, and we're just beginning to realize the extent of the safety crisis in our hospitals.

There are tremendous efforts underway by non-profit organizations and governmental agencies to legislate, entice and cajole the hospital industry into making real improvements. There's lots of consumer advice floating around, urging patients to stand up for their own rights and participate in their own care, but no one seems to acknowledge the difficulty in carrying out that advice. Telling a patient who is frightened, dependent and physically compromised to speak up for herself is like telling a woman in labor to deliver her own baby. It may be possible, but it certainly isn't ideal.

We've become more convinced than ever that bringing a well-prepared personal advocate to the hospital who has no personal interests or loyalties to the health care system is absolutely crucial. The patient needs someone who will look after her safety, make sure her rights and wishes are honored, and speak up on her behalf.

This book provides the inside scoop about how things work in the hospital as well as strategies for leveraging the system, navigating the cultural climate and resisting the internal and external pressure to remain passive about your health care.

We offer practical information that will help patients and their advocates understand:

1. Patient rights, including:
   a. The right to (truly) informed consent. Information on the risks, benefits, alternatives and expected outcomes for any test or procedure must be provided in plain language the patient can understand.
   b. The right to have an advocate involved in all decision-making and information-sharing conversations with health care professionals.
   c. The right to have an advocate present even during invasive procedures, if preferred.
   d. The right to delay or refuse any test, treatment or procedure.
   e. The right to have all pain, regardless of the source, taken seriously and treated aggressively.
2. What questions to ask and what information to document in a bedside chart, and other vigilant behaviors that will significantly decrease the occurrence of medical errors.
3. How to find accurate information about specific diseases, treatments and procedures.
4. How to gain access to the patient's medical record during a hospitalization, and when that would be advised.
5. How to use basic negotiation and conflict resolution tactics to get the patient's needs met.
6. How to choose the battles that really matter and how to carry out effective strategies for winning these battles.
7. How to successfully pre-empt, deflect and defend against retaliation for being "difficult."

We see this book as a gift of empowerment to help patients and their loved ones get what they want and need during a hospitalization, which is always a personal crisis.

If you are the patient, and find yourself alone in the hospital, this book will give you the information you need to be a well-informed consumer, and the tools to advocate for yourself. If you are a concerned loved one of a patient, this book will prepare you to step into the role of advocate and take courageous action on his or her behalf, or on the behalf of any hospitalized individual.

This book also contains an urgent request. Every time we find the courage to insist that the patient's rights are honored and the patient's voice is heard, we have an effect on the system. Please do your part to improve the hospital experience for those who come after you. Sometimes we're patients, and sometimes we're advocates. But always, we're in this together.

Meet the Natives

Understanding the Health Care Tribe

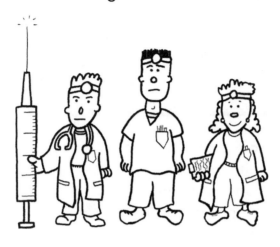

After long careers in health care, we thought we understood the culture because we had insider knowledge about how the hospital works. Then, by some twist of fate, over the last three years the members of our work team – a nurse, a social worker and a healthcare administrator – encountered every aspect of the patient/family hospital experience. These hospitalizations were lived deeply by each one of us as they occurred. When we weren't directly affected, we followed the events closely, offering empathy and emotional support. In this way, we've personally experienced seven Emergency Room trips, nine surgeries, three Intensive Care Unit stays, one birth, and one death.

Now, you should know that the three of us were already passionate health care advocates. We believed in being active participants in our own care and the care of our loved ones. We believed in being vigilant, asking questions and voicing concerns as the front line defense against medical errors. We believed in all the conventional wisdom about the consumer's role in the hospital experience. But we'd never had such immediate opportunities to put our advocacy skills to the test. And the results? Nothing less than shocking.

Steve's Story

I'm one of those guys who takes pride in being a responsible, informed consumer, especially when it comes to health care. So before my outpatient surgery, I went to the Internet to learn what I could do to make sure I had the best possible outcome. Fortunately, I work in health care, so I had access to the most recent scientific studies on best practices. In addition to detailed information about the procedure, I learned that receiving IV antibiotics two hours prior to the surgery drastically reduced the incidence of post-operative infection. Good information, right? So now I've done my part to be an informed patient.

While waiting in the holding area before surgery, I asked the nurse who was starting the IV, "When will I be getting my antibiotic?" She said, "Don't worry, you'll be all right." I repeated my question, and she repeated her answer, "Don't worry, you'll be all right." I quickly discovered that this person's grasp of English as a second language was minimal, so I asked to see the Charge Nurse. As the minutes ticked away, I became more anxious.

Finally, the Charge Nurse came with a frump and a hurrumph and said she would check on my question. After some more hurrumphing and implying that I was ignorant and had no business asking medical questions, she informed me that I wouldn't be getting an antibiotic, because my doctor didn't order it. I inquired further about the presence of standing orders for best practices, and she informed me they didn't have any. Now I'm really starting to get nervous. I asked her to call the doctor and she became visibly upset, saying it wasn't his standard procedure to order an antibiotic. Then she blamed me for not having this conversation with my doctor prior to intruding into their hospital.

I asked to speak with the Charge Nurse's supervisor, who gave me the same story. Finally, I just gave up and went along. I didn't want to make these people mad, because I wanted to get good care. They did finally bring an antibiotic about 30 minutes before surgery. I thought to myself, "Too little too late, or is it better late than never?"

A day after my surgery, I called the surgeon and told him that I was running a fever and couldn't stop shivering, even under an electric blanket. "I think I've got an infection." The doctor said, "You don't have an infection, but I'll give you a round of antibiotics if it will make you happy."

In about two days the "imaginary infection" seemed resolve as my temperature went down and the cold chills stopped. I was weak, angry and frustrated, and couldn't understand why no one would listen to me.

I'm still angry about this. I tried to be a good consumer and got beat up for it. My doctor didn't follow national guidelines to make sure I didn't get an infection. When I got an infection, he denied it and insinuated that I was a crock. It felt to me like a cover up for a medical error. What's going on here?

When Steve shared his story with us, we wondered why the

nurses were so offended by his question, why they were so hesitant to call the doctor, and why the infection that resulted was denied.

Diane's Story

I think the worst part was not knowing what would happen next. My healthy, 56-year-old father had a stroke. We had somehow made it through the ICU part, and the coma part, but when he was moved to a regular nursing unit, he was in between. Not in a coma anymore, but not entirely alert and coherent.

My mom and I tried to stay at the hospital as much as we could, in shifts, but I had young children to care for, and she needed to go home sometime. One morning I went up to see him and found a huge bed outside his room that looked like a cage. When I asked the nurse about it, she said, "That's called a veil bed. We're putting your dad in it so he won't fall and hurt himself. He's been trying to get up all night." I said, "I do not think that will work for our family. Let me call my mom. Are there any other options?"

They didn't like it, but the nurse finally admitted they could move him closer to the nurse's station and install a bed alarm to alert the staff when he was trying to get out of bed.

I couldn't believe they were actually going to put my father in a cage — without even talking to us about it! I imagined that my dad would be absolutely terrified to wake up at night in a cage/tent thing. This certainly wouldn't support his efforts to recover his own independence. We had already offered to come up any time at night, should he need calming down or frequent trips to the bathroom. Still, I did my best to smooth it over. I could tell the staff was not happy that we were trying to be involved in decisions regarding my dad's care. I felt that if they were mad at us, my dad might suffer.

When Diane came back to the office and told us about this we wondered why the nurses would take such a drastic measure without consulting the family, why they were so reluctant to offer less extreme alternatives, and why they were so angry at the family's refusal to go along with their original plan.

Kathy's Story

We really didn't see it coming, because my dad was in relatively good health. He was out shopping all day on Thursday, but Friday morning he woke feeling bad. By the afternoon he was short of breath, and by 10 p.m. we were heading for the ICU.

When my dad agreed to be put on a ventilator because of his severe pneumonia, I asked the doctor in his presence to promise us one thing. "You will keep him sedated, the whole time, right?" The doctor assured us that my dad would be asleep through it all. My dad looked to me for the final decision. "Yes," I told him, with a lump in my throat, "I think this is the right thing to do."

The worst moment came when I walked into my dad's ICU room one morning and found him panic-stricken. His face was a silent scream, his eyes pleading with me to do something. A quick glance at the monitor told me his heart rate and blood pressure where dangerously high.

I ran out to the nurse's station and asked for the nurse caring for my dad. I said, "Please bring something to sedate him. He's awake and agitated, and his blood pressure is through the roof." The nurse looked me up and down. "Impossible. I just gave him something." I was begging now. "Please, just come and see." She followed me. Slowly.

When she saw my dad there was no denying that what I'd said was true. She turned to me and asked a question that still chills my bones. "Do you always have this effect on your father?"

I couldn't even answer. If I started in on her, I knew I might never stop. And I couldn't risk making them angry, because they had my dad! It felt like a hostage situation.

This episode puzzled us most of all. What could possibly motivate a nurse to act in this manner?

Of all the stories we will tell you, these three are probably the most extreme. In each hospital journey we experienced in our personal lives, despite some misadventures and even one significant error, the patient had a good or appropriate outcome. And in each event we were successful in seeing that the patient's most important wishes were honored, thanks to our knowledge of hospital policies and politics. But every single hospital episode over the course of three years left us holding some combination of frustration, resentment and anger on our way out the door. No matter how we approached the staff in our role as advocate, or the relative importance of the issue, we experienced the same emotional storm.

We couldn't seem to avoid offending the hospital staff, and they couldn't seem to avoid offending us. We found this intriguing, because we have three distinct styles: the nurse's way of meeting the health care professionals as colleagues, the social worker's way of affirming the good intentions of the staff and trying to find a solution that works for everyone, and the activist's way of calmly citing patient rights and then accessing the chain of command.

We found our personal "relationship failures" with hospital staff distressing and ironic. As a team, we were being paid to work with hospital staff to improve the experiences for patients and their families! We asked each other many times, "If we have such difficulty as health care consumers, then who doesn't? Does this go smoothly for anyone?" Again and again, the answer was no. We even heard personal health care stories from physicians that are indistinguishable from all the others we've heard.

The questions that plagued us were:
- Why do hospital professionals get so angry when we follow the advice in their own admission materials to speak up, ask questions and participate in our care?
- Why are family members who are also health care professionals treated with suspicion and contempt?
- Why are patients blamed for their own illnesses or bad outcomes?

And the question that haunted us the most:
- Why, despite our knowledge and experience, are we so afraid to speak up for our own family members?

We looked at the situation from every angle. In our work, we paid closer attention to what hospital professionals had to say about patients and family members. In our personal lives, we listened carefully to what friends and neighbors had to say about their hospital experience. We reviewed our own actions and reactions as health care consumers with a critical eye.

For the longest time, our familiarity with the hospital system kept us from seeing the obvious. But when we explored the landscape as amateur anthropologists we started to see a pattern, and then suddenly, everything made sense. **The American hospital has a dysfunctional culture that unwittingly promotes the consumer's feelings of powerlessness and dependency.** Our discovery helped us understand what we had always observed in the behavior of patients, their families and hospital staff. It also explained our own disturbing compulsion to obedience when we were the patients or family members.

We started referring to the "health care tribe," because so much of the behavior reminded us of tribal customs that are unspoken, maybe even unconscious, and extremely resistant to change. When we use this term we are not implying that health care professionals are primitive. We are just describing the unique features of their culture. If you think about it, tribal behavior seems to be hard-wired into our genes. You will see it everywhere like-minded humans gather: professional societies, urban gangs, churches, social clubs and playgrounds. All tribes have a membership rite, a hierarchy of status, unspoken rules about acceptable and unacceptable behavior, a special language, and a distrust of outsiders.

The big difference is the amount of power the health care professionals have over patients and their families. The educator's tribe has the power to give you a bad grade, and the real estate tribe has the power to diminish the profit on the sale of your house, but the hospital tribe has the ultimate power. They hold our personal comfort, health and well-being in their hands.

Navigating this dysfunctional culture would be challenging in the best of times. Unfortunately, we're more likely to arrive at the hospital when we're at our absolute personal worst. A combination of physical distress, anxiety, and maybe even white-knuckled fear, does not put us in any position to make clear-headed decisions or reasonable requests.

The moment we find ourselves in that vulnerable position of needing health care, something strange happens. We revert to childhood, when mother magic could make it all better. No matter how bold or assertive we may be in ordinary times, suddenly we want to be told what to do. Any negotiation skills we have are put on hold, or somehow come out in a twisted, aggressive way. Our response to vulnerability will vary from individual to individual, but one thing's for sure: we are in a position of dependence, and we know it. We're in a perfect state to follow the nearly irresistible urge to become a "good patient" or a "wonderful family member," which is exactly what the hospital culture wants us to do.

When we assume the role of good patients and wonderful family members, we defer to the experts and do as we're told. We are in awe of the caregivers and intimidated by our surroundings. We don't question the natives' judgment or ask for excessive explanations. We try very hard not to "waste" the natives' time, and when we make requests or ask questions, we are appropriately apologetic. We show the natives at every opportunity that we know our place.

We behave this way because we are very, very afraid. We are afraid for our health, or the health of our loved ones, and we believe that if the natives like us, we'll get better treatment. We're afraid of making our caregivers mad, and we're afraid to even imagine what the repercussions might be. The hospital culture exerts subtle, and sometimes direct, pressure to reinforce that fear.

Amazingly, the majority of hospital professionals are not consciously aware of this. They don't notice the unequal balance of power and the unspoken burden of fear that is deeply felt by the patient and family. The natives truly believe that all we have to do is speak up if we've got a problem. They don't notice that when we do just that, they label us as "difficult." Once that label is pronounced, there is a chance that the staff will change their behaviors towards the patient and family. This can be terribly unpleasant and might include withholding information, or slow responses to requests for pain medication.

We believe the natives don't notice the patient's fear because they're too busy battling their own. Fear of errors, lawsuits, licensing boards, doctors and supervisors creates an incredibly stressful work environment and explains most of the dysfunctional behavior. Quite possibly, the natives are even more afraid than we are, and their fear is pervasive, unrelenting and contagious.

Don't be discouraged by what we're telling you. Five or maybe 10 years from now, things will be very different. Change is in the wind. Lots of internal and external pressure is being exerted to transform the old culture, making the hospital system more inclusive of the patient and family. One day, in every hospital in the country, you will encounter health care professionals who are eager to listen to you, include you in planning your care and empower you with your decision-making rights. And it will be the norm, not the exception, as it is today.

But for now, the best approach is to enter the hospital the same way you enter a foreign country. Expect difficulties, inconveniences and miscommunications. Be vigilant. Plan ahead for every contingency and have a well-prepared advocate at your side.

This travel guide will assist you on your journey. The advice and strategies we offer directly result from our breakthrough discoveries regarding the hospital's culture and the hours we've spent listening to Traveler's Tales, the stories of patients, family members and advocates. If you can find the courage to put these tools into practice, you will have a safer, more comfortable hospital stay, with the best possible outcome.

CHAPTER 2

The Rules

Unspoken Rules of the Health Care Tribe

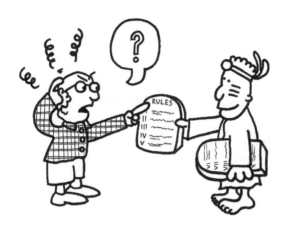

I. The Natives are in Control
II. The Natives are Experts
III. Power is Distributed Through the Chain of Command
IV. The Official Language is "Medical-eze"
V. The Official Currency is Time
VI. "Normal" is Defined by Tribal Standards
VII. The System Serves the Masses
VIII. The Natives are Paranoid
IX. Enemies of the Tribe are Punished
X. Failure to Recover is an Insult to the Tribe

I. The Natives are in Control

As soon as you sign on the dotted line of your admissions papers, you are a ward of the system. The natives are responsible for your health, and they take that charge very seriously. You have become a liability to them. Everything that happens to you while under their care is documented and potentially reviewed. Each time they document something in your chart, their license and credibility is on the line, not just for today, but until the statute of limitations runs out. There are lots of rules, and lots of reasons for all the rules, but the natives don't feel compelled to explain them. They want to control what happens and leave as few decisions to you as possible. Their control is a carefully guarded commodity, and if you try to capture a little corner of it, they will let it be known that you are difficult.

Traveler's Tales

My husband likes to be in control. The first thing he does when he steps foot into a hospital is to bend the rules. If they try to put him in a small room with obviously sick people, he'll refuse to wait there for health reasons. If they tell him to take off his clothes, he'll only do it under duress. Even then, he might keep on his pants. If they tell him to sit in a chair, he'll say, "I prefer to stand." If they tell him to lie on a stretcher, he'll sit in the chair.

The smart ones just let him have his way, and then he mellows and becomes more cooperative. But usually, his antics reduce health care professionals to a quivering rage. And they retaliate by labeling him as "difficult." You wouldn't believe how fast that label travels through the grapevine, making each interaction with a new staff member more unpleasant than the last.

Every time, I find my husband's behavior embarrassing, and I defend the hospital staff for trying to enforce the rules. Still, it amazes me how inflexible they are, especially when these small acts of defiance don't amount to a hill of beans.

Failure to fall into the good patient or wonderful family member role results in being labeled as difficult. This label has unpredictable but inevitable repercussions, based on the tactics of individual staff members to correct the problem behavior. News of a "difficult" presence spreads through the hospital faster than a virus.

Note: If you're into control in your regular life and can't keep yourself from exerting it under every circumstance, expect a bumpy ride in the hospital.

Survival Tips for Rule #1
A. Choose your battles wisely.
B. Be a good guest and observe the rules when it doesn't matter that much.
C. When the rules interfere with the best interest of the patient:
  1. speak up,
  2. do it respectfully, and
  3. move up the chain of command.
D. Take a pro-active stance to deflect the "difficult" label.
  1. If you're the patient, blame/lean on the advocate.
  2. Deflecting blame to the advocate allows the "good patient" label to stick.
E. Disprove the rumor.
  1. Turn on the charm.
  2. Prove your reasonableness in other matters.

II. The Natives are Experts
You can safely assume that the professionals providing your care know what they're doing. Every health care license requires initial training, a rigorous exam and lifelong continuing education. From doctors and nurses to respiratory therapists and dieticians, they're all required to keep their knowledge and skills up to date. They all have to answer to a code of ethics, and there are serious consequences for sub-standard practice.

That's the good news. The bad news is that when you combine

Rule #1 and Rule #2, you have experts who want total control. This leads to a paternalistic "father knows best" attitude towards patients. Often, the option that seems best to them is the only one they'll tell you about.

Traveler's Tales

I've learned to be suspicious when a doctor or nurse says, "If he was my father, I'd want him to (fill in the blank)." I always think, "But this isn't about your father. It's about my father and his situation at this particular time. Besides, I don't even know if you like your father!"

Experts are generally terrible listeners. When we try to tell them things we know about our own bodies, or what we know about our loved one's situation, they either cut us off or endure our explanations with glazed eyes.

Traveler's Tales

Every time I bring my mother to the hospital, which is quite often, we go through the same routine. I tell them that they're going to need a pediatric needle to start the IV. They never listen. After several sticks they get the pediatric needle, and sure enough, it works. This is hard on my mother and hard on me, but what can you do?

Experts do not like having their skills or judgments questioned. They do not like to be told how to do their job. You will be labeled as difficult if you insinuate that your family member is getting poor care, or that the natives don't know what they're doing, especially if you do it five minutes after you arrive.

Traveler's Tales

Eight hours after my c-section delivery, a nurse came into my room and said, "Up, up, up! I want to see you walking down the hall to that nursery!" I obediently hauled myself out of bed and staggered down the hall, depending heavily on a flimsy IV pole. The Charge Nurse saw me, ran over and asked, "What do you think you're doing? You shouldn't be out of bed yet!" I tried to tell her about the other nurse, but she would hear none of it. I got a good scolding all the way back to bed. Later I learned that the "nurse" who flushed me out was actually a nurse tech, a high school graduate with a bit of on-the-job training.

There are lots of patients in hospitals, and lots of staff members wandering around in similar outfits. Mistakes happen. If you are asked to do something or go somewhere, and you haven't been prepared to expect it, throw a flag on the field. You nearly always have time to find out more. If someone comes into your room and announces, "Time for you're electroshock therapy," and it's the first you've heard about it, just say no!

Survival Tips for Rule #2
A. Don't assume you're talking to an expert.
   1. Always, always, always read name tags — know who you're talking to!
   2. If you're instructed to do something that doesn't make sense, ask to talk to a nurse.
B. When dealing with experts:
   1. Listen to what they say.

2. Ask questions.
3. Ask about alternatives.
4. Keep asking questions until you understand.
5. Educate yourself.
6. Ask if they have information you can read.
7. Search the Internet. (See Appendix D: Surfing for Answers.)
8. Ask different health care professionals the same questions and compare answers.

C. If you need to convey important information that will impact care:
1. Tell them what you know politely, but firmly.
2. Take another health care professional's name in vain.

> Examples:
>> "The last time I needed an IV, they had to call an anesthesiologist. He said this vein is the only hope. Would you mind trying this one first?"
>> or
>> "My mom's doctor said to be sure and tell you..."

3. Refuse the treatment or procedure and move up the chain of command until someone listens to you.

D. If you have doubts about a staff member's competency:
1. DO NOT allow them to touch you or your loved one.
2. Ask to speak to the Nurse Manager; voice your concern and ask for someone else to be assigned to your care.
3. If that's not successful, ask to speak to the Nursing Supervisor.

III. Power is Distributed Through the Chain of Command

Every hospital has a hierarchy, and the patient is at the bottom of the ladder. Next comes the clerical staff and technicians, and then the professionals. All of the professionals have a direct supervisor, or manager, and a director responsible for the entire service. Generally, nurses rule, but they have a hierarchy as well. A staff nurse provides the bedside care, a Nurse Manager is in charge of the unit, and the Nursing Supervisor oversees all. Next, there's the Director of Nursing, or Chief Nursing Officer, and then the Hospital Administrator. After hours, there is always an administrator on call.

The chain of command rules the hospital, and there are two chains. Doctors run the medical care, but they don't run the hospital. Usually they are not hospital employees. Hospital admissions, treatments, procedures and medications require a doctor's order. They have a great deal of power, because without them there would be no hospitals. Everyone jumps when the doctor barks, from the hospital staff to the executives in the boardroom.

Survival Tips for Rule #3

This rule can cut both ways, but in the hands of a committed advocate, it can serve the patient very well.

A. Never let the staff use the hierarchy against you.

Refuse to accept the following "reasons" for delays in your treatment or changes you've requested in your care:

1. "We don't want to wake the doctor."
2. "My supervisor's not here."
3. "Your doctor always/never wants things done this way."
4. "Let's just wait and sort this out tomorrow/Monday."

B. Use the chain of command to your advantage.

1. Try to resolve any problems at the point of care.
2. Make sure you're talking to the person who can make it happen.
3. Never hesitate to go directly to your doctor; call the office number if necessary (this number is answered 24 hours/day).
4. When it really matters, scale the chain of command: Charge

Nurse to Unit Manager to Hospital Supervisor to Administration.

5. Access the hospital's internal advocacy resources: talk to the people who are skillful at working the chain of command for you. You'll find these people in the departments of guest relations, social work, patient advocate or ethics.

6. When you exhaust internal resources, go to external ones (see Chapter 9 for contact information for Medicare, Joint Commission for Accreditation of Health Care Organizations (JCAHO), your insurance plan, etc.).

IV. The Official Language is "Medical-eze"

Every expert culture has its own language. The language of medicine is hard to understand, but when it's peppered with abbreviations and slang, it can sound like word salad.

The natives have been speaking their language for so long they don't even notice it. They honestly believe they are communicating with you in English! A delightful minority can translate into English without being prompted, but the majority has to be asked for definitions and clear explanations.

Many of us endure this gibberish because we're worried about looking stupid. Some of us write down the word salad and pour over medical dictionaries to try to figure out what they said. This is an unnecessary burden. You do not need to take a crash course in medicine to get good care! Our vocabularies naturally expand when we're involved in our own health care, and we're all free to do as much outside research about our particular situation as we want. Still, the health care professional has a responsibility to educate us, and we need to hold them accountable to this responsibility.

Survival Tips for Rule #4

A. Know the patient's rights regarding communication with health care providers.

1. The patient has the right to understand every aspect of his/her care.
2. The health care professional is obligated to provide information that the patient or the patient's agent can understand.
3. If the patient's language of choice is not English, the health care provider is required to provide professional translation services (in person or via telephone).

B. Insist on understanding what you're told.
   1. Whenever you hear a word you don't understand, ask them to explain it in plain English.
   2. Repeat your understanding back to them, to make sure you got it right.
   3. Write it down, and write down the health care professional's name, also.
   4. If the response you get is less than favorable, politely remind them of the patient's rights regarding communication.
   5. If you're still not satisfied, move up the chain of command.

V. The Official Currency is Time

Managing time is very difficult in hospitals, because there is so much unpredictability. When the natives have plenty of time, they still act as if they have none. They don't know what's going to happen in the next minute or the next hour, so they guard their time as a precious commodity. Taking up less time than usual makes you a good patient. Taking up more time than usual makes you a difficult patient. The same standard applies to family members.

Traveler's Tales

The first night I was in the hospital, the pain became absolutely unbearable in the middle of the night.

I tried to just tough it out because I didn't want to bother anyone. Finally, I couldn't stand it any longer and I called the nurse. "You're going to have to call the doctor and wake him up. I've just got to have something for this pain." The nurse said, "Oh, you have pain medication ordered. I'll bring it to you." Why didn't they tell me about that? I suffered for no good reason!

The time management tactics of the natives seems to consist of silently chanting the mantra, "no time, no time, no time,", and rushing through everything as if the place were on fire. This makes patients and family members feel guilty for every request, because it seems to take the staff away from other Really Important Things.

Traveler's Tales

When my husband was in the ICU after a brain hemorrhage, I waited patiently for an opportunity to talk to the doctor. I had so many questions! When I finally cornered him, he said, "I don't have time to talk to you. If I talked to all the families, I wouldn't have time to take care of patients, now would I?"

After that, I just talked to the nurses. But all I really got was, "He's doing as well as expected." I never tried to talk to the doctor again, because I felt guilty and embarrassed for bothering him.

Family members are generally seen as time wasters. The natives get especially frustrated when they have to give the same information to various relatives. The family gets very frustrated when they compare notes and come up with different stories.

There is a new tactic being used by staff, and occasionally by doctors, to keep from having to deal with family members. HIPPAA, the federal Health Insurance Portability and Accountability Act, has established new standards to safeguard the "confidentiality, integrity and availability" of electronic health care information.

This has resulted in a new push for better confidentiality of medical information in general. Patients should be asked on admission for the names of people who can have access to information about their condition. If a family member is not on the list, (or if the health care professional doesn't bother to consult the list, or doesn't even make a list), they will hear, "In order to protect the patient's confidentiality, I am not at liberty to talk to you about his/her care."

Survival Tips for Rule #5

A. Ask for what you need.
 1. Don't let the frantic pace of the staff keep you from asking for things you really need (i.e. pain medication).
 2. Don't expect the staff to tell you everything about everything. They believe it's your job to ask. So ask!
B. Endear yourself to the staff.
 1. Acknowledge their time constraints.
   a. "I know you're very busy, but would you mind ..."
   b. "When you have a chance, could you ..."
   c. "I hate to bother you, but I need help right away ..."
 2. Offer to operate on a "self-serve" basis.
   i.e. "My sister needs a cup of ice and a blanket. If you'll show me where it is, I'll be glad to get it for her."
 3. Remember the boy who cried "Wolf!"
   When you save "I need you right now" for times when you really do, you're more likely to get what you need in a timely manner.
C. Talking to the doctor is a necessity, not a luxury.

1. Be prepared. Keep notes of the questions you have, and record the answers.
2. Don't be intimidated.
   a. Let the doctor know you intend to be involved as a part of the team.
   b. If your doctor won't talk to you or partner with you, get another one (see Chapter 4, Who's Driving This Bus?).
3. Set expectations.
   a. Inform your primary care physician, or the primary specialist, that you expect him or her to act as captain of your health care team.
   b. Ask when you can expect a daily update from this doctor; offer options (in person, phone calls, e-mail).
   c. Ask about daily goals and the goals for the hospitalization.
   d. Track test results and record them.
   e. Insist upon informed consent.

D. Make a family communication plan.
   1. Appoint a family spokesperson.
      a. Choose someone who is a reliable, effective communicator.
      b. This person should take responsibility for keeping everyone else informed.
   2. Get hip to HIPPAA.
      a. Keep a list of the people who should be informed about the patient's condition, signed by the patient.
      b. Let the doctor and staff know who needs to be involved in decision-making conversations; share the patient's list if there is a question.

VI. "Normal" is Defined by Tribal Standards

In the hospital, normal is pretty strange. Imagine if part of your daily tasks at work was putting tubes and needles into people. After a while, it would seem normal, right? To health care workers, probing your body is an everyday thing. It doesn't occur to them that it's about as far from real world "normal" as it can possibly be.

The best health care professionals carefully explain what they intend to do, make sure you understand, get your consent, and comfort you along the way. Others don't bother. They do these things so often; it hardly seems worth a mention.

Traveler's Tales

A nurse came into my dad's room in the Emergency Department and started laying out a bunch of tubes and needles on a tray. He didn't introduce himself or explain anything. Right before he stuck the needle in, he said his first and only words. "Brace yourself." I was furious! When I asked my dad what he thought about it, he said it didn't bother him a bit. He said, "I knew what he was doing." I couldn't believe the total lack of respect.

Really invasive, even permanent assaults on your body are also seen as routine, if not normal.

Traveler's Tales

The doctors and nurses occasionally mentioned in an off-hand way that they'd probably need to perform a tracheotomy, because the tube that goes down the throat and connects to the ventilator is very irritating and can cause serious damage after a couple of weeks. The idea of our dad with a temporary, or possibly permanent, hole in his throat was a huge deal to us.

We knew that he would absolutely hate it.

The doctors and nurses couldn't understand our revulsion. A nurse actually said to us, "It's really not a big deal." My immediate mental response was, "It's not a big deal for whom?"

Another side effect of this distorted view of normal is a frequent failure to adequately prepare the patient for procedures or treatments.

Traveler's Tales

They said they were going to do a bone marrow biopsy, so I thought, "O.K., it's like a lab test." I've never had such blinding pain in my life! If I had any idea that it would hurt so much, I would have demanded sedation.

Pain, unfortunately, is way too "normal" in the hospital. There is a certain amount of discomfort and pain that goes along with receiving treatment and getting well. But there is always medication available to diminish, if not relieve, any pain.

Traveler's Tales

My husband's number one priority in the hospital is to be prepared. He can take nearly anything, as long as he has a minute or two to process it. No matter how many times he explains this to health care workers, they just don't get it.

During the infamous kidney stone incident, someone just appeared by his stretcher and announced, "Time for your CAT scan!" As they wheeled him down the hall, I heard him protesting, "What CAT scan? What's this all about?"

By his report, when he got to X-ray a nice woman explained that she'd be giving him an enema with contrast media. When he got even more upset she said, "Oh, they didn't tell you?" (According to my husband, she said it like this happened a lot.)

When I met up with him again after the test he said, "If somebody did that to me out on the street, I could press charges!" And you know what? He's right.

Informed consent means you've been informed of the risks, benefits, alternatives and possible outcomes. Performing invasive procedures and tests without informed consent is technically considered battery, and it's illegal.

Tying people down in the hospital used to be normal, but not anymore, thanks to consumer activists in the mental health community. Wrist restraints are fairly common to keep patients from pulling out their tubes, and vest restraints are used to keep people from climbing out of bed. There are tons of rules that have to be followed when it comes to restraints. A doctor has to write the order, it's only good for 24 hours, and the restraint has to be released hourly to check circulation and to make sure it's still needed. The family has to be notified as well. If restraints are really necessary for the patient, the advocate should make sure they're removed the minute they're no longer needed.

Survival Tips for Rule #6
A. Don't take anything for granted.
1. Know before you go.
   a. Don't go anywhere, with anybody, unless you know: who, what, why, when and how.

DON'T GO THERE ALONE!

b. If the staff insists, just dig in your heels and say you need to talk to the doctor first.

2. Write down names and titles. If you can't read their name tags, ask them to tell you who they are and what their credentials are.

3. Question the use of restraints.

    a. Let the staff know that the family or advocate should be notified if restraints are recommended.

    b. Ask for less extreme safety measures.

    c. Ask the staff to remove the restraints whenever the advocate or family is present.

    d. Voice any concerns to the doctor.

B. Ask, Ask, Ask

1. Before any treatment, test or procedure, ask for a thorough explanation of what you can expect.

    a. What type of preparation is required? Do I have to drink something, stop eating and drinking for hours before, etc.?

    b. What will happen during the treatment, test or procedure?

    c. How will I feel during and after?

    d. When will we have the results? Who will tell me?

2. Before any treatment or procedure, ask if there will be pain.

    a. Expect them to minimize the pain you will experience.

    b. Don't fall for euphemisms, such as "discomfort," "sting" or "pressure."

    c. If the treatment or procedure involves pain, insist on pre-medication.

    d. If you're denied pre-medication, remind them of the JCAHO regulations mandating the patient's involvement in the care planning process, including the plan for pain management.

C. Find out the word on the street. Talk to someone who has first-hand experience.
    1. Ask the health care professionals if they've ever had this done.
    2. Ask them what patients usually say about the experience.
    3. If there's time, ask your peers in the hospital, ask among family members and friends, or do some research on the Internet (see Appendix D: Surfing for Answers).
D. Insist on adequate preparation for discharge.
    If you'll be leaving the hospital with less or more than you came in with, make sure you understand how to manage at home.
    1. Make sure you know how to manage any tubes, treatments, procedures or new medications.
    2. If you leave the hospital with less function, even temporarily, make sure you know what to expect and what type of assistance you might need.

VII. The System Serves the Masses

For all the talk in the official public relations material about individualized attention, hospitals are organized for large-scale health care delivery. The hospital system is designed to deliver health care to the masses, generically saving lives and stamping out disease.

The natives look at patients as an anonymous whole. Their focus is portioning out care from highest to lowest need, accomplishing tasks, and completing documentation. Their work is smooth when the patients are "good" (i.e. obedient) and the families are "wonderful" (i.e. docile). Patients blend together, except for the ones who are very sick or "difficult." The natives see individual needs and requests as barriers to doing their jobs. The whole system is threatened when family members ask too many questions and patients make too many requests. "Too many" is a number known only to the tribe.

So there is a natural conflict of interest between us and them. We are focused on obtaining the best possible care for ourselves or our loved ones. The health care professional is focused on providing the best possible care for everyone. Our objective is the same, but our focus is different.

Traveler's Tales

Sometimes I'm absolutely convinced that health care is run by 18-year-old girls. There's always one at the front desk, and if I didn't know there were trained people in the wings, I'd be really worried.

I took my mom to the hospital for a mammogram one year, and the technician (an 18-year-old girl) looked at her, eyed her wheelchair suspiciously and then said, "Honey, can you walk ... at all?" My mom politely told her no, but the girl wouldn't drop it. "Can you stand up ... or anything?" Again, my mom told her no. The girl didn't try to hide what a huge inconvenience this was for her. I kept my mouth shut, because my mom is the "good patient" extraordinaire.

The next year, we returned. Same time, same place. The technician (another 18-year-old girl!) looked at her, eyed her wheelchair suspiciously and said, "Honey, can you walk ... at all?" My mom politely told her no, but she wouldn't drop it. "Can you stand up ... or anything?" Again, my mom told her no.

I had a nearly irresistible urge to say, "Honey, I personally haven't seen this woman walk since 1978, but now that I think of it, you're probably right. I'll bet she can walk! I'll bet she's just been messing with us!"

I'm sure these girls have no idea what effect they have on patients. But it's certainly clear that they see any modifications to their well-oiled machine as a huge inconvenience.

Even though the hospital is required to make accommodations for individual needs, they're not very good at it. It disrupts their business and alters the flow of work.

Traveler's Tales

The stroke has left my wife with serious, permanent problems. We recently spent nine hours in the Emergency Room, and it was a nightmare. I had to make them change her adult diaper. If I hadn't been there, it would never have occurred to them. And no one even thought about feeding her!

When they discharged her, the doctor said, "You can take her out through that door." I asked, "You want me to take her out through the waiting room and put her in the car in front of all those people?" He said yes. "Do you realize that she's naked from the waist down? When I give you back your sheet, there's going to be quite a show." And this was a hospital!

Survival Tips for Rule #7

A. Enlist the help of your doctor.
   If the doctor orders it, it has to be done. (That's why they call it an order!) If you need some special modification to the way things are normally done, you doctor can make it happen.
B. Stand on the patient's rights.

When you're told that modifications for personal needs aren't possible, tell it back to them.

"So you're telling me that there's no way my mom can have a bath in the evening instead of in the morning? Isn't the bath a part of the care plan, and isn't it the patient's right to be involved in planning that care?"

C. Negotiate.

  1. Find a way to get what you want and allow them to save face (for detailed negotiation strategies, see Chapter 9, There's a Fly in Her Soup).

  2. Offer to go on the self-serve plan.

    "I'll be happy to bathe my mom every night. Just show me where the supplies are."

VIII. The Natives are Paranoid

Health care is a highly regulated system. Violating rules and failing to meet standards of care can have dire consequences for the hospital and the natives. Health care professionals have licenses they fiercely protect.

The fear and paranoia of the tribe stays at a manageable level if the patient and family members are sufficiently ignorant. Those who have educated themselves are assumed to be dangerous by the tribe, so they imply that any consumer knowledge is probably misinformation. The natives love to shroud everything in mystery and keep family members or advocates away from the action. Witnesses make them very nervous. They will tell you that it's in the best interest of the patient, but it's really in service to the comfort of the staff.

Traveler's Tales

The minute my dad heard he needed a heart

catheterization, he asked if I'd be there with him. He was so proud that I'm a nurse, and saw it as a perk that he had one for his very own whenever the opportunity presented. I told him to ask his doctor. The doctor had no problem with it, so we arrived the morning of the procedure and I asked the nurse where I needed to go to gown up. She stalled, saying her supervisor needed to talk to us.

The supervisor arrived and said, "My staff doesn't feel comfortable having you in the room. There could be complications, which would be very hard for you to watch." I tried to negotiate with her, telling her that I would be respectful of her staff and even promising to leave the room any time they asked. The supervisor said, "You don't understand. Bad things could happen. It could get messy. You could see things you don't want to see. If it was my dad ..."

I cut her off to keep her from scaring my dad anymore. "Fine. Fine, I won't go in." My dad jumped in and said, "Yes, I know bad things could happen. That's why I want her with me." The nurse just turned up the gas. Her descriptions became more graphic of all the terrible things that could happen until I surrendered. "Fine!" I practically screamed. "I already said I won't go." Finally, she was satisfied.

Then I said something that proves how intimidating the situation is, even for health care professionals. "I respect your professional judgment." So, not only were we bullied and terrorized by this nurse, I thanked her for the abuse!

The Emergency Nurses Organization has officially taken a

position in favor of family presence during invasive procedures and resuscitation, but this is not commonly accepted in hospitals. The patient has the right to have an advocate or loved one at their side in most situations, and studies have shown that it benefits the patient and family. Even if the patient doesn't survive, the loved ones have less complicated grief, with the comforting memory of being with the patient through it all. But making it happen takes committed and determined advocacy.

Health care professionals from other tribes are treated as interlopers who know too much. The natives will not be impressed if you bring your own expert. If you have a family member who is a doctor or nurse, or if you are a doctor or nurse, you will set yourself apart as someone to be cautiously dealt with. The non-native expert will need to proceed with caution to avoid serious clashes (unless, of course, a serious clash is the only possible way to get the patient what he or she needs).

Traveler's Tales

I don't like health care providers to know that I'm a nurse. Nurses, especially, seem threatened. When my family members are in the hospital and need an advocate, they proclaim loudly and often that their own personal nurse is on the way. When I show up the staff makes me feel as welcome as Typhoid Mary.

The natives are brave in the face of illness, disease and life-threatening events, but they're very afraid of regulatory or accrediting agencies, and they are absolutely terrified of lawyers.

Their lawyer phobia will cause them to assume a lawsuit is in the works if the family requests a copy of the chart, takes pictures of anything, or asks too many probing questions.

Traveler's Tales

When my father-in-law was in the hospital after surgery, he had a horrible time getting pain management and basic care. The family kept calling me because I'm a nurse. I coached them long distance and finally just said, "Ask for a copy of the chart." They did, and immediately his care improved. I hated to do that, but there didn't seem to be any other way to get their attention.

Mistakes and errors affect human lives with serious personal and tribal consequences. The tribe's response is to admit nothing, deny everything, and make counter-accusations, blaming the patient if necessary.

Traveler's Tales

My mom came out of surgery with a terrible sore on the inside of her nose. When I asked about it, they mumbled around and finally said it was caused by pressure from a tube during surgery. It took forever to heal, and she almost had to have plastic surgery.

I've since learned that this was a mistake. They're supposed to protect the patient from this type of injury and, obviously, someone wasn't paying attention. But they tried to pass it off as something that just happens.

You have the right to know if a mistake or "unanticipated outcome" has occurred during your care. Currently, the doctor is only required to inform you if a serious, irreversible mistake happened (this is called a sentinel event). But if you get an explanation about why there's been a change in your care that doesn't make sense, or if the health care professionals seem to be secretive or avoiding your questions, ask your doctor.

Survival Tips for Rule #8

A. Insist on disclosure.
1. Let the doctor know that you expect honesty and that your continuing relationship depends upon it.
2. Find out how the mistake impacts the patient's care and treatment, and what to expect during the recovery.
3. Ask why a mistake happened and how they plan to make sure it doesn't happen again.

B. Avoid frightening the natives.
1. Advocates or patients who are also health care professionals should tread very lightly; your credentials will hang over the situation like a very big stick.
2. Threatening legal action while you are currently a patient is a risky proposition. You will get attention (lots of it!), but it sets up an extremely adversarial situation.

C. When necessary, use their paranoia to your own advantage.
1. Calmly cite JCAHO or Medicare regulations, or read from the list of patient rights that was given to you at admission.
2. Anything you do that implies you might be thinking of legal actions will bring on a flurry of activity on your behalf. You will be suspect and could be labeled an enemy of the tribe, but you will see action.
3. Suggested activities include asking to see the chart, asking for a copy of the chart, taking pictures of the "problem" or asking to talk to someone from the Patient Safety or Risk Management departments.
4. If you've tried every other remedy, and feel calling your lawyer is your only recourse, don't announce it. Just do it.

D. Don't become infected with their paranoia.
  1. Even though paranoia is hanging in the air, don't fall victim to it. Refuse to be bullied, refuse to be intimidated, refuse to be discouraged from doing the right thing. They're more frightened than you are.
  2. Be realistic about your care. A less than desirable outcome doesn't mean someone is at fault.

IX. **Enemies of the Tribe are Punished**
  Enemies of the tribe fall into two categories.
  1. "difficult" patients and family members
  2. lawyers, or those who associate with them

"Difficult" patients and family members come in all shapes and sizes. Usually, the label is attached when you ask excessive questions, insist on modifications to the natives' routines, or complain about care. If you are a Very Important Person, either out in the world or according to hospital administration because of some inside ties, you are already teetering on the edge of difficult. The health care tribe has a very socialistic attitude toward patients. The only difference is in how sick they are. Nothing chafes a native more than being told that a patient is a V.I.P., and there could very easily be a backlash, just to take them down a notch or two.

There are definite repercussions for being difficult. Your antics will be passed from shift to shift during report. In no time at all, everyone in the place knows that you are "difficult." The staff may be colder than usual. They might not laugh at your jokes. One or two of them might let a catty comment slip out. If it's very important to you that the whole world thinks you're wonderful, this might be hard to take. Even if you're fairly thick-skinned, minor slights can be more irritating than usual when you don't feel well.

Repercussions can be more serious, like delays in getting your pain medication, withholding information or restricted visiting in intensive care. If you feel serious repercussions are occurring, the advocate needs to act and act quickly.

If you work for a lawyer, if your husband, wife, brother, sister, mother or father is a lawyer, or if by some terrible chance you are a lawyer, guard this information with your life. DO NOT let the natives know about this "unsavory" aspect of your character.

Patients and their family members are afraid of causing problems for the staff, because they worry it will affect their care. No matter how "difficult" you are, the vast majority of health care professionals will strive to deliver the best care possible, even to jerks, lawyers and those who consort with lawyers.

Survival Tips for Rule #9

A. Avoid being labeled an enemy of the tribe.
  1. If anyone implies that you're difficult, you have two options.
    a. Disprove it immediately.
    b. Go full out, high velocity "difficult" and make the most of it.
  2. If you have a close relationship to a lawyer, or if you are one, don't let them know. If they find out, ingratiate yourself to them; compliment them and let it be known that you are not at all like most lawyers, or their close associates. You're just CRAZY about health care workers and think all this lawsuit business is downright un-American.
B. If you are labeled as an enemy, use the tribe's paranoia to your advantage (see Survival Tips for Rule #8, The Natives are Paranoid).
C. Defend against retaliation.
  1. Talk to your doctor about your fears. In this situation, your doctor isn't just your best friend; he or she may be your only friend.

2. Recognize the signs.
   a. Slow response answering call lights or requests.
   b. A sudden insistence on rigidly following "the rules."
   c. Withholding information or dispensing it tersely.
3. At the first sign of retaliation, put the staff on notice.
   a. Let the Charge Nurse and Nursing Manager know that retaliation has occurred and will not be tolerated.
   b. Ask to speak to the patient advocate/guest relations representative or a social worker, and report what has happened.
4. Flee from the offended party.
   a. If you're considered an enemy by one staff member, ask for the assignment of a different staff member to provide care.
   b. If you're considered an enemy by the entire nursing staff, ask to be transferred to another unit.
D. Resist the pressure to be "good."
   1. Don't let the fear of being labeled "difficult" keep you from asking for what you want or need.
   2. Let the advocate be "difficult" for you.
   3. Remember:
      a. You may never see these people again.
      b. Your health is more important than the "Congeniality" award.
      c. There are worse things than being labeled (like spending the night in a cage bed!).

Note: If you are extraordinarily "difficult," or if you threaten legal action, the hospital can put you on a "do not admit" list. If your name is on this list, they will not admit you to the hospital again unless your life is in danger. This is not necessarily a bad thing. If you feel you have to be excessively "difficult" to get the care you need, you should find another hospital anyway.

X. Failure to Recover is an Insult to the Tribe

Blame is an incredibly pervasive part of the health care culture. You may be blamed for your condition, especially if your unhealthy lifestyle choices landed you in the hospital. You can pretty much expect to hear, "This is what you get for smoking," or "Your diet is killing you." Usually, we're already blaming ourselves.

You may also be blamed for not responding to treatment. The health care tribe is in the rescue business, saving lives and stamping out disease. It's particularly ludicrous to blame the patient for failing to recover, but it happens all the time.

Traveler's Tales

When my dad was in ICU, every couple of days someone would ask me again about the history of his illness. I always told them the same story: He was out shopping the day before. He woke up the next morning feeling bad. He took a nap in the afternoon, and when he woke up, he had trouble breathing. He went to the doctor and was sent home with antibiotics. I took him to the ER around 10 p.m., and he ended up in ICU.

About two weeks into our ICU stay, a nurse we were particularly fond of came up to me and said, "Your dad didn't tell you the truth. He was sick for days. He couldn't be in this condition now without being sick for days. He should have gone to the doctor sooner." This young man was visibly angry! I think he was angry because my dad just kept getting worse, and he needed someone to blame.

Since that happened, I've paid more attention to this illogical "blame the patient" phenomena, and it's surprisingly common. When my husband went in for a hernia repair, the first thing the nurse said to him was, "You shouldn't pick up heavy things and then you wouldn't need surgery."

It is important to understand what caused your problem if it's possible to modify your behavior and avoid a repeat of your current situation. But knowledge and blame are distinctly different. Blame is delivered in a tone of voice that implies, "Don't expect sympathy from me when this whole thing is your own fault." Blame has a tendency to give you a sense of shame and a sick feeling in the pit of your stomach.

Along with blame, denial is rampant in the hospital when patients fail to recover. Remember, many health care professionals, including doctors, consider death a personal insult. Studies show that aggressive care in Intensive Care Units often continues even when there's no hope of recovery. Doctors say they do this for the sake of the family, but just as often, they probably do this for themselves. To break bad news to someone, first you have to break the bad news to yourself.

Traveler's Tales

I remember the moment when I first tried to talk with the doctor about my father's wishes regarding life-sustaining treatment. When he had an episode of very low oxygen levels despite the ventilator, I told the doctor about my father's advance directive. He'd even taken the trouble to deliver it personally to the hospital a couple of years earlier, after suffering a severe heart attack. The doctor said, "I think it's too early to talk about this."

My dad depended on me to advocate for him, and I

wasn't going to let him down. I said, "If his heart stops, he wouldn't want you to perform C.P.R." The doctor again said, "It's too early to talk about this." Somehow I restrained myself from asking, "How could it possibly be too early to talk about an advance directive?" Instead, I asked, "If his heart stops, even though he's on a respirator, that would be a very bad sign, don't you think? If his heart stopped, and you got it going again, what would be the odds that he'd ever walk out of here?" The doctor reluctantly admitted that the odds were practically nil.

The nurses got the word about the "Do Not Resuscitate" order the doctor wrote, and they cornered me in the hall. "We just want to make sure what you're asking for. Do you want us to stop all treatment?"

How could this be so foreign to them? I assured them we wanted my dad to continue getting treatment; we just didn't want a full blown code if his heart stopped.

Later, a nurse said to me, "We're not giving up on your dad." Another pulled my brother aside and told him, "I don't know what your sister is talking about. Your dad is doing just fine!" I had committed the unforgivable sin of initiating the conversation about the possibility that he might not recover.

Eight days later, the last day of my dad's life, I told the lung specialist that we didn't want my Dad put back on the ventilator. He looked at me grimly and declared, "I don't give up on anyone." I'd had enough. I looked back at him with steely resolve and said, "You know what? This isn't about you. And it's not about me. This is about my dad. And it's my job to tell you what he'd tell you if he could talk."

It makes me sad, and worried, that those nurses and doctors didn't realize how much they added to our burdens. I wonder if they learned anything, or if they're still slinging guilt at family members to this day. But I did my job. It was the hardest thing I've ever done, and I'm really proud of myself. For once, I had the courage to stop trying to please them and make them like us. I focused on my dad, and that's all that mattered.

Survival Tips for Rule #10:

A. Don't accept blame.
  1. If you are the activist type, let them know you find this offensive.
  2. Otherwise, just let it go.
B. Ask for a family conference with the doctors.
  1. Insist that a time is chosen when everyone can be there.
  2. Feel free to ask for family time alone during the conference to talk privately.
  3. Keep your focus on the patient. The doctors are experts, but the family is the expert on the patient's wishes.
C. Help them tell you the truth, by asking:
  1. What are the goals now? How have they changed?
  2. What do we know? What don't we know?
  3. What are the chances the patient will walk out of here?
  4. What is the benefit of what we're doing (tests, monitoring, treatments)? What is the burden? What would happen if we just stopped?
D. Insist that the patient's wishes are honored.
  1. Make sure the doctor and the nurses have a copy of the advance directive.
  2. Even without an advance directive, in most states the legal

next of kin can speak for the patient and make decisions according to their understanding of the patient's wishes, or what the patient would say if he or she could speak.

3. If you feel the patient's wishes are not being honored, consider a change (different doctor, different hospital, going home).

E. If the illness is life threatening, or recovery is in question, ask for a palliative care or hospice consult.

1. Palliative care is the management of pain and symptoms.

2. Hospice care is a redirection of goals from cure to comfort. Palliative care and hospice care nurses and doctors are excellent advocates, who will help evaluate the need for burdensome treatments and help the patient and family design a plan of care that is appropriate, with a focus on the quality of life.

3. If the doctor or staff resists, insist.

The Company You Keep

Building A First-Class Health Care Team

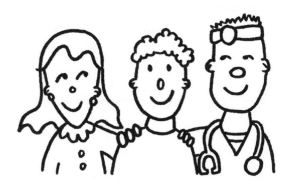

If you were going to a foreign country, you probably wouldn't just throw yourself at the mercy of random people and hope for the best. Most likely you would complete an extraordinary amount of research, because you want to have the best trip possible, and you want to be safe.

Researching your health care choices is even more important. Choosing wisely will have an enormous impact on your health care experience. It's not an exaggeration to say that your life may depend on it.

Finding a Primary Care Physician

Finding a physician who a) fits your definition of a good doctor, b) is on your health plan, and c) practices in your hospital of choice can seem like winning the lottery. But it should be your highest priority. Preferably, you should line up this doctor when you're relatively well and have the energy it takes to sort through all your choices. Your primary care physician should be someone you feel comfortable with, someone you trust, and someone who respects your wishes. If your current doctor doesn't fit this description, find another one.

Ask around. When you hear someone say they've been to the doctor, ask them for the name and if they were satisfied with their experience. People love to talk about their health care experiences. Ask your hairdresser or barber; they probably hear more medical stories than should be allowed. If you know any health care professionals, ask them who they would choose for a primary care physician.

After you've gathered a few names and crossed off the ones that aren't on your health plan, your next step is basic research to verify training and competence. Even though medicine is a noble profession, doctors are people, and people tend to fall somewhere on the bell curve. Ten percent are very, very good at their chosen profession, and 10 percent are very, very bad. The rest fall somewhere in the middle.

Look for a doctor who is board certified in Family Practice or Internal Medicine. This certification tells you that the doctor went through specialized training and passed a rigorous exam, in addition to his medical school training. It also indicates that his knowledge is current, because certification has to be renewed every seven to 10 years, depending on the specialty. If the doctor advertises that he or she is board eligible, this doesn't really tell you much. A doctor can be board eligible for years and never pass the test.

It's not a bad idea to see if they've received any disciplinary action from their state medical board. Some states make this information available to the public, while others don't. Check out your state medical board website (www.fsmb.org).

Serious consumers want to know about malpractice cases against a doctor, thinking this will be the best way to weed out that bottom 10 percent. It's certainly a red flag if the doctor is involved in multiple malpractice cases, but guilt cannot be assumed until the case is resolved, and that can take years. Malpractice settlements don't reveal that much either. Insurance companies will settle claims just to be done with them, even when the doctor probably would have won the case. But disciplinary action is a very bad sign that probably should eliminate that doctor as a choice. You may choose to make some allowances for administrative infractions, such as not releasing medical records in a timely manner, but it's still a red flag.

After verifying the basic competence of the doctor, you'll want to meet him or her in person. Some doctors will set brief appointments to meet perspective patients for no charge, while others charge for the visit. This is kind of like a blind date. All you'll really get is a first impression, which could turn out to be wrong. Still, you have to start somewhere.

The place to start is with you. You'll be most successful finding a good fit with a doctor if you're able to take an honest look at what you really want in this relationship. Based on your personality, past experiences and expectations, do you want a doctor who is:

- professional or personable,
- serious or light-hearted,
- attentive to the details or more concerned with the big picture, or
- a father figure or a partner?

No one is perfect, so you have to set priorities. If it's really important that your doctor has a first class education and an impeccable reputation, you may have to accept her poor listening skills. If you need a doctor who will really listen and spend his office time generously with you, you'll need to pack a lunch and bring a book to your appointments, because he'll probably treat other patients the same.

You may not even be able to identify what you want in a doctor, but you'll know it when you see it. That's why the doctor-shopping visit is so important. You can get a feel for the doctor, the office staff and the general atmosphere of the practice.

Ask the doctor about:

1. Philosophy of care: the answer to this question will give you an idea of how the doctor carries out his practice. Listen for clues regarding style.

2. Communication: Will you be communicating through the nurse? What are the nurse's credentials - RN, LVN/LPN or nursing assistant? (This makes a huge difference in the weight you give to the "nurse's" advice.) Does the doctor have a certain time each day for returning calls? Is e-mail communication a possibility?

3. After-hours availability: What should you do if you have a problem in the evening or during the weekend?

4. Partners: Are there other doctors in the practice who might be responsible for your care during the doctor's absence? Are they board certified?

5. Hospital affiliations: If the doctor practices at more than one hospital, ask which hospital she prefers for her own health care needs.

6. Hospital practice: If you are admitted to the hospital, will this doctor still be involved, or will your care be handed over to others? Is the doctor willing to serve as the captain of your health care team, regardless of the problem or number of specialists?

7. Referrals to specialists: Does the doctor refer to a specific group of specialists? Is the doctor open to your own investigations and choices?

8. Opinion of complementary therapies: How does the doctor feel about other therapies that are important to you, such as herbal remedies or chiropractic care? Share any interests or

preferences you may have in this area and take note of the doctor's response.

9. Sharing information: How does the doctor feel about routinely mailing your test results, so you can maintain your own personal medical records? How does the doctor feel about disclosure of errors or poor outcomes in your care? It's a good idea to let the doctor know your expectations. Do you want an honest relationship, even when it comes to bad news? Or do you prefer that the bad news goes to your advocate first?

Pay close attention to how the doctor talks to you and treats you. Do you feel comfortable with this person? Trust your instincts. If you don't find the right doctor on the first try, just keep trying. It's worth a great deal of effort to find a doctor in whom you have confidence. Then you can build a relationship of trust, which is absolutely priceless.

Choosing a Specialist

When you are referred to a specialist by your primary care physician, it's important to remember that doctors are also running a business, and the medical business depends on referrals. You could be referred to a mediocre specialist because he or she recently sent several patients your doctor's way. Always ask for two or three names, and don't be shy about asking your doctor which one is the best. Then carry out the same research that led you to your primary care physician, including the shopping around visit.

Finding a Hospital

Investigate the reputation of hospitals in your area. The Joint Commission for the Accreditation of Healthcare Organizations (JCAHO) is an independent, not-for-profit organization that evaluates the quality and safety of hospitals through a regular survey process. The survey results of participating hospitals are listed on their website. You can also call JCAHO's Customer Service Department directly at 630-792-5800 for additional information. The Centers for Medicare and Medicaid Services (CMS) also posts patient satisfaction scores for hospitals, and you can compare the scores of hospitals in your area.

If you know any health care professionals, ask which hospital they'd choose for themselves or their family members. They're more likely to know the inside scoop.

Call the hospital's main number and ask to speak to someone in administration.

Find out:

1. Is the hospital a designated trauma center? If so, they will have specialists available to respond to emergencies anywhere in the hospital.
2. If it's a small hospital, ask how they handle transfers to larger hospitals when a patient's needs are greater than the hospital's capacity. Ask to which hospitals they most often transfer their patients. Investigate those hospitals as well, to make sure they are acceptable choices for you and your family.
3. Do they employ intensivists, doctors who specialize in the care of patients in Critical Care Units? Studies have shown that outcomes are better for patients who are cared for by intensivists.
4. Do they have a pain management team in the hospital? Pain that is difficult to manage is a serious problem, and having experts available makes a big difference.

When you're in the neighborhood, it's a good idea to go into the hospital and just mill about. Notice how you're greeted. See how people are behaving in the waiting areas, especially in the Emergency Department. In general, do they seem fairly content, or are they agitated? Sit for a few minutes and eavesdrop. What happens when they ask the staff questions? How are they treated? Does the staff wear name tags that you can read? In a short time you can get a feel for the place. Is this somewhere you'd choose to go if you were sick?

Choosing Your Advocates

We have already established that when you're the patient, you're severely handicapped when it comes to exerting power on your own behalf. In theory, all health care professionals promote the role of advocacy. It's part of the professional obligation of doctors, nurses and social workers to advocate for you. Every hospital has employees whose time is at least partially dedicated to the patient advocate role. While these people can be very helpful, you still need your own advocate who has no personal interests or loyalties to the health care system. You may need several advocates, depending on the situation and your level of stress. Consider the roles of the advocate.

Companion

There's a lot of waiting involved in health care. It is very comforting to have someone to keep you company when you're feeling bad or anxious.

Navigator

In many hospitals, it's very difficult to find your way around. When you're already stressed, it's a lot easier to get lost. Having someone with you helps a lot.

Recorder

Physical and emotional distress can affect what you hear and understand from your doctor and other health care professionals. The advocate can take notes about tests and procedures, treatment options, medication changes and instructions. You should spend your time listening, not writing.

Representative

When you fall into the "good patient" routine, your advocate can speak up for you, making requests, asking questions and insisting on getting you what you need.

Mediator

At times you may need someone to give you a reality check. You may get very upset or antagonistic because of your own internal turmoil. Your advocate can help you choose your battles.

Spokesperson

Sometimes when you don't feel well, just talking to friends and family can be a burden. Your advocate can provide updates on your condition and answer any questions, according to your wishes.

Safety Monitor

There is always a need for vigilance in the hospital. The number of patients who suffer injury and even death from medical errors is under debate, but we know for sure that it's a problem in every hospital. Patients are much less likely to get the wrong procedures, tests and medicines if someone is paying close attention and asking questions.

Junk Yard Dog

Occasionally it is necessary to become assertive when dealing with health care professionals. Your advocate can do the hard work of insisting that your rights are honored, moving up the chain of command and registering complaints on your behalf.

When Do You Need an Advocate?

- When you're anxious about an office visit to a physician.

- When your doctor is explaining test results or planning for any medical or surgical treatments.
- When you're meeting with a specialist.
- Anytime you go to the hospital, for any reason.

Who Qualifies as Your Advocate?

Your primary advocate should be your closest relative or closest friend. You will need secondary or emergency back-up advocates for times when your primary advocate is not available.

Advocate Qualities

The very best advocate is someone who has training in advocacy and conflict resolution. Formal training would be ideal, but the information in this book can help prepare anyone to advocate for you. The best choice is someone who possesses the following qualities:

- assertiveness,
- good communication skills,
- grace under pressure,
- confidence in the face of authority, and
- a strong stomach.

If you know someone like that, you're really lucky. If you know someone like that who also loves you madly or owes you a tremendous debt of gratitude for past good deeds, you've got it made! If such a person doesn't exist in your life, settle for someone who is willing to go with you and able to hold your hand. Any port in a storm.

Preparing Your Advocates

In order to have the best possible outcome, you need to know your rights and wishes, make sure your advocate knows your rights and wishes, and agree on a plan to make sure they are honored.

Understanding Your Rights

1. You have the right to a clear understanding of everything that happens, and to be provided with all the information you need to make decisions about your care.
2. You have the right to know the name and credentials of everyone involved in your care.
3. You have the right to have your pain taken seriously and treated aggressively.
4. You have the right to privacy and confidentiality.
5. You have the right to include anyone you wish in information-sharing or decision-making conversations with health care professionals.
6. You have the right to have your wishes honored for appropriate and medically indicated care, or if you want to be transferred to another facility.
7. You have the right to question anything and everything.
8. You have the right to say no.

You are the ultimate decision maker. This includes deciding who can speak for you when you find it difficult or impossible to speak for yourself.

Establishing Your Wishes

It is important to review your expectations every time you put your advocate to work. For a doctor's appointment you might need help writing down what the doctor has to say and remembering the questions you want to ask. If you're going to the hospital, make sure your advocate knows your general wishes about your care. For example, you will want your advocate to be with you before and immediately after surgery. You may want them to protect your privacy, gently shooing away acquaintances that come by to visit. It's important that you spell out what you expect them to do.

Because it is impossible to plan for all of the situations that could come up during a hospitalization, you may need to ask for time alone with your advocate to discuss new treatments or decisions you're facing. Take this time as situations are presented. These private conversations will allow you to specify, based on new information, any actions you'd like the advocate to take on your behalf.

Your advocate also should know your wishes regarding life-prolonging treatments in case you are diagnosed with a terminal condition (not a pleasant topic for discussion, but still necessary). A Living Will is the preferable way to accomplish this. The Living Will helps your advocate remember what you want and lets the health care provider and other family members know your wishes as well, in case your advocate's instructions are challenged.

Appointing Your Advocate
Informal Appointment:
1. Bring your advocate and introduce them to the health care professional as your advocate.
2. Make it known that your advocate will stay with you during any discussions of your condition and treatment. You can request that your advocate stay with you during treatment as well.
3. Make sure that your advocate's name and contact information is listed on your chart.
4. Make sure that your advocate is designated to have access to all information regarding your condition and treatment. (There may be a section of your chart for this information. If not, ask the health care professional to write it in.)

When Do I Need to Make a Formal Appointment?
The law in most states makes provisions for health care decision-making when you are unable to speak for yourself. Particulars vary, but legal power is granted according to relationship. Usually if you are married, your spouse can make those

decisions. If you are single, in most states, the majority of your adult children are legally able to make decisions for you. If you're single without children, the rights go to nearest relatives. If you have doubts that your next of kin will agree to support your wishes, it's very important that you legally name someone you trust for this responsibility. Even if your legal next of kin is your first choice, it's a good idea to legally appoint them as your advocate (sometimes called agent or proxy) so there will be no doubt of your intention that this person speaks for you. (See Appendix C: Traveling Papers.)

How Do I Make a Formal Appointment?

Health Care Power of Attorney (also called Health Care Proxy): In this legal document, you can designate your advocate as your decision-maker if the situation ever occurs that you are unable to make decisions for yourself. This capability will extend to times when you are sedated, unconscious, or unable to make your own decisions because of temporary or permanent loss of mental function. This is hard core advocacy, with an incredible amount of responsibility. You should have complete trust in this person, and they should have complete understanding about your wishes.

Before you hand over that kind of power, ask yourself if this person has the courage to put your needs and wishes above everything else, including the desire to be liked and the fear of embarrassment. Ask yourself: If push came to shove, could this person throw a public fit on my behalf?

If choosing and preparing your advocate sounds like a big job, you're right. But planning ahead by carefully grooming your advocate, along with cultivating a really good relationship with a primary care physician you completely trust, will radically improve your chances of getting the very best medical care with the very best possible outcome. It's your health and your life. What could be more important?

CHAPTER 4

Who's Driving This Bus?

The Patient's Role and the Advocate's Mission

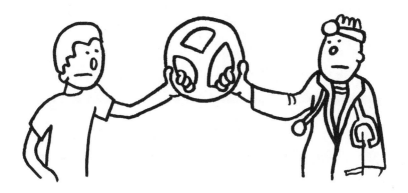

The Patient's Role

When you're the patient, you don't need advice; you need real help. Even though the advice in this book is practical and tested, it's still advice. In order to best turn this advice into real help, we recommend that you:

1. resist the "good patient" fear of making the health care tribe mad,
2. be completely truthful with your advocate, and –
3. let your advocate go to work for you.

Asking someone to be your health care advocate is a big deal. Consider making an advocacy pact: "I'll do this for you, if you'll do this for me." Knowing that you will return the favor should the opportunity present itself will make the advocate's personal sacrifice on your behalf easier to bear.

The Mission of Advocacy

Serving a loved one in the role of health care advocate is absolutely an act of love. It's normal to approach the task with anxiety, especially if you don't have a lot of experience or knowledge in health care. We don't want to minimize the difficulty, but we want you to know that anyone can do this. You don't have to understand medical words or procedures, change your personality, or neglect the responsibilities in the rest of your life.

Advocating for a loved one requires:

1. understanding the needs and wishes of the patient,
2. collecting and sharing critical information,
3. being present at a critical moment,
4. a willingness to ask questions,
5. a commitment to stand up for the patient, no matter what, and
6. recognizing when you're in over your head, and calling in reinforcements.

(Remember, as an advocate you are not there to practice law, medicine or other professions. Do not hesitate to contact the appropriate professional for advice and assistance.)

Patient Advocacy in Four (not so easy) Steps
1. Be Prepared

There are some things that every patient needs, including pain relief, appropriate and timely treatment, informed consent, basic respect and comfort. Then there are specifics that you, as advocate, need to know.

- You need to know about dietary needs and any individual requirements for the patient's sense of comfort and security.
- You need to know the patient's medical history.
- You need to know the names and phone numbers of everyone who should be informed about the patient's condition.
- You need to know the name and phone number of the primary care physician and any specialists involved in the

patient's care.

- You need to know about, and have a copy of, any Advance Directives (see Appendix C: Traveling Papers). If the patient doesn't have Advance Directives, you should strongly encourage completing them, even helping to fill them out, if necessary.
- You need to make sure the patient designates you, in writing, as someone who has access to their confidential medical information so you can participate in the health care team, taking part in discussions, asking questions and gaining access to the patient during care.

2. Be There

Every patient should have an advocate at their side:
- throughout an Emergency Department visit,
- during admission to the hospital, from the business office through the initial nursing paperwork, until the patient is settled into the room and comfortable,
- during decision-making discussions with doctors, from the time immediately before surgery or other invasive procedures through the initial recovery period, preferably for the first 24 hours,
- any time the patient becomes confused or agitated from medication or disease, or
- during discharge discussions with nurses and doctors.

3. Speak Up

As a general rule, you should ask questions any time you, as an advocate, don't understand what is going on, or if it's obvious that the patient doesn't understand. Asking questions can make the patient very nervous. Don't be surprised if the patient asks you to back down and just go along. It's helpful if you can talk about the "good patient" syndrome in advance and find out what the patient wants you to do before they actually become a patient. If you're really clear about what you've been charged to do, it's easier to just blast away with the questions, ignoring the patient's efforts to "make friends" with the health care provider.

If it becomes necessary, moving into full-blown patient advocacy will make the patient nervous for sure. Again, if you know what you've been charged to do, it's a little easier. But only a little.

Insisting on the patient's rights will not win you many friends in the hospital. When you stand up for the patient, you break the unspoken rules, and the staff can't just stand by and let that happen. They might make you feel like a troublemaker and a busybody. They might make you feel ignorant. They might make you feel like you have committed a deadly sin. To be a good advocate you have to ignore all of this and stay focused on the patient. It takes courage.

We have found it helpful to give ourselves pep talks in the middle of the storm.

"I'll never see these people again."

"No one has ever died of embarrassment."

"I'm not here to win a popularity contest."

"The squeaky wheel gets the grease."

"If I don't speak up now, I'll always regret it."

(For specific actions and strategies, see Chapter 9, Speaking Out, Speaking Up.)

4. Get Help

Patient advocacy shouldn't be a marathon; it should be a relay. It's really hard, emotional work, and trying to do it all yourself is just asking for disaster. If you don't get enough sleep or spend enough time taking care of the details of your own life, you'll be a less effective advocate. It's very important to put some time and thought into building your support system before you become exhausted.

Talk to the patient about friends and relatives who want and need to be involved. When people say, "If there's anything I can do," be ready to hand them an assignment. People really do want to help, but don't know what's needed. Try to coordinate their visits to get the most bang from your resources. At the very least, someone should visit the patient each day. Ideally, the patient should have someone with him or her when the doctor visits; before, possibly during, and after invasive procedures; and whenever a change is made in the plan of care.

It's hard to anticipate when these things will happen. Hospitals are notorious for running on their own timetable and failing to properly inform the patient's family. As the advocate, you can improve the chances of staying informed by making a habit of stopping by the nurse's station and reminding the staff that your phone number is on the chart and you expect to be called if there are any changes. You should also remind the doctor, in person or through notes left at the bedside and with the nurses, that you expect regular updates in person or by phone. If the doctor and the staff get into the habit of calling you when necessary, you can relax a little. Over time, if you are able to establish this trust, you'll be able to take care of your own needs without being so worried.

Remember, even though advocating for a patient in the hospital is stressful, it doesn't last forever. It's a wonderful, priceless gift that radically improves the patient's chances of getting the very best health care and the very best outcome.

CHAPTER 5

Point of Entry
The Emergency Department

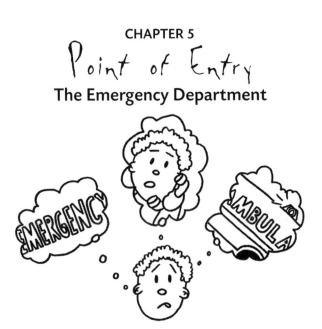

TO GO OR NOT TO GO

The Emergency Department is the place to be when there is significant or continuous bleeding, severe pain or shortness of breath, sudden change in mental status, loss of consciousness (even for a short time), or sudden inability to walk.

You certainly need medical attention if you think you've broken a bone, if you have a deep cut that obviously needs stitches, or if you have distressing symptoms that won't let you rest until the morning. Actually, you need medical attention anytime you think you need medical attention! It's always better to be safe than sorry. But does that medical attention have to come from the Emergency Department of your local hospital?

The important word here is "emergency." Going to the Emergency Department for the treatment of a sore throat is like going to a five-star restaurant for a grilled cheese sandwich. You can certainly get it there, but it's going to cost you. When you arrive in the Emergency Department of a hospital, the first person you will encounter will be the triage nurse. Triage means "to sort." After a quick once-over, the triage nurse will categorize your complaint as an obvious emergency, a strong potential for emergency, a potential emergency, or a non-emergency. Some hospitals have a "fast track" process to move the sore throats out quickly, but if seriously injured people arrive, everybody waits while the life-threatening issues are addressed.

You might consider a "doc-in-the-box" minor emergency clinic or waiting to see your primary care physician if:

- your problem has been going on for days or weeks,
- you know you need to see a doctor, but there's no real sense of urgency, or
- you need care, but not full blown emergency care.

Insider's Tip: For "non-emergency" emergencies, plan your arrival for times when the Emergency Department is likely to be slow. Usually, things are relatively quiet from midnight to 10 a.m., and very quiet from 1 a.m. to 5 a.m. Most people come when it's convenient for them and their companions: after lunch, after school, at the end of the work day, or after their evening meal. The best possible time to go is during the Super Bowl, and the worst time is immediately after the Super Bowl! Going in the middle of the night is inconvenient, but will significantly decrease your wait time.

GETTING THERE

Calling an ambulance

If you have a true emergency, just call 911. Sometimes it's just a judgment call, but if you think you might be having a heart attack or a stroke, calling 911 is the only reasonable course of action. You should know that once the ambulance guys show up, you're pretty much at their mercy. Don't assume you know your destination hospital. The ambulance crew has the authority to take you to the nearest hospital if your condition is considered life-threatening. Or, if your neighborhood hospital happens to be swamped at the moment, all ambulances can be diverted to other hospitals. Have your advocate follow the ambulance to make sure you both end up at the same place.

Traveler's Tales

When I broke my heel, the pain was unbearable, so I asked my co-worker to call 911. I'd fallen from a very tall ladder, so I really didn't know how badly I was hurt. The paramedics got there pretty quick, but when they checked me out, they seemed disappointed that I wasn't bleeding or anything. When I asked them to turn on the sirens and hurry up, they flatly refused. And I was paying for this!

Insider's Tip: Paramedics tend to be adrenaline junkies. They'll probably be disappointed to find you a good distance from death's door. Try to overlook any bad manners; it's just a ride, but it's a ride in a rudimentary rolling hospital (which is a really good place to be if your physical condition is shaky).

GETTING THERE BY PRIVATE CAR

If you're sure it's not a life-or-death emergency, you can go to the Emergency Department by private car. Have someone drive you, or take a cab. Do not drive yourself. Even if you're feeling fine, you may be given medication that will make it unsafe for you drive home. If you drive yourself, you'll have to park, and you may have quite a hike to the Emergency entrance. (If it's not a big deal to walk a mile or two from your car, you probably don't need to be there. Go to a minor emergency clinic or wait to see your primary physician in the morning.)

Traveler's Tales

My mom couldn't breathe, so I panicked and just threw her in the car and raced to the hospital. Looking back, it was a very risky thing to do. What if she'd lost consciousness? What if she'd died in my car? Why didn't I just call an ambulance?

Insider's Tip: When in doubt, call 911. If you over-react, you can live with that. If you under-react, you will be very sorry.

WHAT TO BRING
If you have a little time and presence of mind, bring:
- insurance/health plan card,
- list of current medications,
- picture identification,
- credit card or checkbook,
- pen,
- change or small bills for vending machines, and
- something to read.

If you are on medications that need to be taken at certain times, bring them with you. The Emergency Department does not usually dispense medication unless it's directly related to the situation at hand.

Dress is "come as you are." The Emergency Department staff is accustomed to dirty, disheveled and inappropriate clothing. Don't spend time spiffing up (you'll probably never see these people again).

GETTING IN
How you get in depends on how you arrive and the seriousness of your condition. If you arrive by ambulance, you will be taken directly to a treatment room. If you come by private vehicle, you'll stop by the triage desk. If you are in obvious distress, you'll be taken directly to the back. Otherwise, you'll wait.

Because of strict federal laws that prohibit discrimination when patients don't have insurance or money, most hospitals won't even ask for financial information until you've been seen for a brief medical exam. If you have a true emergency, they have to treat you. They will certainly bill you later and even send you to a collection agency, if necessary.

WAITING

Pay no attention to the order in which patients are seen. The sickest get treatment quickest, no matter how long others have been waiting. Remember, this is not a restaurant! Proper E.D. etiquette involves going where you're told to go and waiting patiently. Waiting is an unavoidable part of the process. Even if you're taken to the treatment area immediately and seen by the doctor, there probably will be lab work, X-rays and other tests. All these tests have to be ordered, performed, processed and interpreted, and that takes time.

You will wait. You can wait the easy way, or you can wait the hard way. The easy way involves amusing yourself. The hard way involves getting angry and demanding, which will brand you as "difficult."

Still, patient waiting should fly out the window under certain circumstances. Your advocate should make your needs known, especially if you are hungry, thirsty or need help going to the bathroom. Your advocate should always alert the triage nurse if you are in severe pain, if you feel like you need to lie down, or if you think your condition is getting worse. All that waiting doesn't happen in a vacuum, and you should be re-evaluated if your situation changes. They actually have a word for this. When they take your vital signs again while you wait, they say you've been "re-vitalized." (If only it were true!)

Traveler's Tales

My 4-year-old son had bronchitis and started gasping for breath about bedtime. I took him to the Emergency Department and we waited a couple of hours. His breathing gradually calmed down, so I just took him back home and waited for the doctor's office to open the next morning.

Insider's Tip: If you discover that you're really O.K., and the wait is incredibly long, you can leave without being seen. Just because you've signed in doesn't mean you have to see it through to the bitter end.

AMUSEMENTS

Usually there is a television in the waiting area, and usually it's tuned to some daytime program you wouldn't watch if someone paid you.

During normal business hours, the hospital gift shop and cafeteria might serve as tempting amusements. Send your advocate on any out-of-the-area expeditions so you don't lose your place in the process. If you feel you simply must leave the area, tell the admissions clerk and get back as fast as you can.

Insider's Tip: Do not eat or drink unless the nurse says it's O.K. Most Emergency Departments have a policy that no one eats or drinks until they have been seen by the doctor. There may be tests that require an empty stomach. If there's any chance you might need surgery, there's a risk that stomach contents will get into the lungs during anesthesia. Who wants to run the risk of getting pneumonia, or even dying, from a candy bar you ate out of sheer boredom? If you're hungry or thirsty, send your advocate for what you want, and as soon as you get the "all clear," you can have it. Gum or hard candy can see you through until then.

GETTING TREATMENT

Finally someone calls your name or number, and you advance to the treatment area. If the natives are very busy and all the rooms are full, you may be parked on a stretcher in the hall. This is just fine, because you're objective is to get in, get seen and get out.

BRING YOUR ADVOCATE WITH YOU!

He or she may be asked to step outside to protect your privacy during examinations, but there really isn't any reason your advocate can't stay with you most of the time, or all of the time, if you wish. Ask you advocate to keep notes for you. They should record staff members' names, which will come in handy if you need to relay what someone told you to another staff member. Your advocate should also write down what the doctor says to you. This is a stressful time, and you may not remember it all later.

Insider's Tip: One advocate or companion should be sufficient; two at the most. It really riles up the staff if a large crowd of people try to come back to the treatment area. There's not a lot of space, and the natives get testy if they can't move freely about the room. If you are especially well loved, or if you are very sick and people want to come and see you, it would be better to wait until you leave the Emergency Department. If you want to see more than one person, they need to take turns.

A nurse or tech will take your vital signs again, and then a physician will come to examine you. If lab work is ordered, someone will come and draw your blood. You may be taken out of the department by wheelchair to other departments for tests. If so, put your advocate in charge of your valuables! Thievery is not unknown in the hospital.

If you leave the department for other tests, your advocate can go with you. Sometimes patients have to wait in dimly lit hallways or windowless rooms in the bowels of the hospital for considerable chunks of time. This is never a pleasant experience, but it's much worse if you're alone.

Insider's Tip: For any test or treatment other than a lab draw or a simple X-ray, always, always, always ask: is this going to hurt? Numbing your skin before inserting an IV or giving you a mild sedative before a mildly traumatic test takes time and may not be offered if you don't ask for it. So if you're skittish about this kind of stuff, be sure and ask.

When all the test results are in, the doctor will give you a "best guess" diagnosis and map out a treatment plan. If the proposed treatment seems extreme, such as surgery, other invasive procedures or a transfer to another hospital, ask the E.D. doctor to call your primary care physician to discuss the plan, even if it's in the middle of the night. Your personal doctor is the captain of your health care team, and important decisions always require his or her input.

GETTING OUT

There are two ways to get out. You could be admitted to the hospital or discharged to the wide world again. If you are admitted to the hospital you could still have a wait, because you won't be able to leave until someone is free to take you to your room. There will be more paperwork to fill out, including a list of your personal belongings. Any valuables should be turned over to your advocate. The hospital probably has a rule that they must secure your wallet and jewelry in their vault.

If you are discharged you may get a prescription to take home and a referral to a physician for follow-up. The nurse will give you written discharge instructions; make sure you clearly understand what you're supposed to do. You'll have to stop by and sign some papers and arrange payment with a clerk. This is a perfect time to ask them to fax a copy of your medical record for this visit, including all test results, to your primary care physician. (If you have the doctor's fax number with you, it's more likely to happen.) And then you're on your way.

Traveler's Tales

My dad saw his primary care physician a few hours before we went to the Emergency Department. On his sixth day in ICU, my mom ran into the doctor in a hospital corridor. We thought it was kind of strange that we hadn't seen him, but it was a pretty chaotic time. Imagine our surprise when we learned that he had no idea my dad was in the hospital!

NOW YOU'RE OUT! BUT YOU'RE NOT FINISHED YET ...

Make sure your primary care physician knows you were in the E.D. Call the office first thing in the morning, even if you're admitted to the hospital. When you call, be sure to mention any prescription medications you were instructed by the E.D. physician to take. If your records weren't faxed, ask the office staff to get copies from the hospital, and ask them to mail you a copy. This becomes an important part of your personal medical record. (You can request copies of your records directly from the hospital medical records department, but they're easier to get from your doctor. Requesting records for your own information gets the natives' paranoia going, and they can make it hard for you.)

CHAPTER 6

The Day Trip

Outpatient Surgery and Procedures

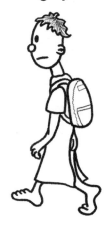

At the Time of Scheduling

Make sure you understand why your doctor is ordering this procedure or surgery, what the risks and benefits are, and what alternatives may be open to you (see Appendix C, IV: Informed Consent). Ask for a business card from the doctor. Be sure to ask about how your discomfort or pain will be managed. If the doctor expects that you will have pain in the hours or days after the procedure, ask if you can fill the prescription the day before (this will keep you from pacing in the pharmacy on the way home, making a spectacle of yourself and frightening random children).

It's important to remember that your surgery or procedure is no big deal to the health care tribe, because they do this every day (remember Rule #6: "Normal" is Defined by Tribal Standards). You may have to really probe to get information about what to expect in the days and even weeks after your surgery or procedure. Commonly, the pain, discomfort and impact on daily life is minimized by the health care professionals. They may have no idea what it's really like, because they're not the patient! They may not even hear about it, because most people don't call in to complain unless things are really bad at home, and the doctor doesn't see the patient again until he's fully recovered.

It's a good idea to talk to someone who has lived through the experience. Ask the doctor if someone on his staff could call a "recovered" patient, and then give them your number and ask them to call you. Ask around among your friends and acquaintances; maybe somebody knows somebody who's been through it. Even though this seems like a lot of trouble, having realistic expectations will make it easier to prepare mentally and to line up the help you'll need as you recover.

Before You Go

Some hospitals and health care centers have online pre-registration; others do it by phone or ask you to stop by. It's good to get this out of the way, so you don't have to worry about filling out forms on the day of your procedure.

Make sure you're very clear about the preparations, and follow the instructions to the letter. Not doing this can mean your diagnostic studies have to be repeated. If you eat or drink the morning of surgery, you will be at risk for aspirating stomach contents into your lungs during anesthesia. If the staff finds out, your surgery will be cancelled. If you keep it from them, you're taking a big risk. It's in your best interest to always strictly follow the pre-operative or pre-procedure instructions.

At pre-registration, if you're not offered a map of the facility, ask for one. Make sure your advocate knows exactly where to park, which entrance to use and where to go for check-in. When you arrive that morning, you don't need the extra stress and confusion of wandering around aimlessly at the risk of being late.

What to Bring

Wear loose, comfortable clothing, which will make it easier to get dressed when it's time to go home. Bring two or three pillows to make the trip home more comfortable. Waiting for your procedure to begin can be excruciating, especially if the natives are behind schedule (which you can expect). You'll be thirsty, hungry and nervous. Bring something to occupy your time; a book, a portable CD player with your favorite music, or whatever will serve as a good distraction for you.

Leave your contact lenses at home, and bring a container for dentures, removable dental appliances or hearing aides. It's best to leave your purse or wallet at home and give your identification and insurance cards to your advocate to carry, along with the doctor's business card.

Getting Started

After announcing your arrival, you'll be taken to a preparation area. The nurse or assistant will come in and ask questions about your medical history. This is the time to produce your personal information sheet, which should include most, if not all, answers to the questions. This sheet should also list any special needs you might have, the name of your advocate, and contact information for family members who have your permission to access your medical information (see Appendix C,II: Letter to all Health Care Providers; and Appendix C, III: Medical History and Personal Information).

During this first interview you'll be given some information about what to expect. Feel free to ask questions, and encourage your advocate to ask questions as well. A patient identification bracelet will be attached to your wrist. Look at it carefully; make sure your name is correct, and make sure any allergies are clearly listed on the band.

If the surgery or procedure involves anesthesia, you'll meet your anesthesiologist or nurse anesthetist. (An anesthesiologist is a doctor, and the nurse anesthetist has been through a rigorous post-graduate anesthesia course. One is not better than the other; experience counts more than anything.) This person will ask another battery of questions and then examine your mouth and neck if your procedure will be done under general anesthesia, which requires a breathing tube while you're "out." Be sure to declare any dental work. Broken teeth, crowns or bridges can occur during general anesthesia!

During this preparation period, your doctor should at least pop in and talk to you briefly. If you're having surgery, your doctor should mark the site so there's no possibility of confusing left and right. This is the time to remind the doctor of any special concerns or requests. Ask about the doctor's plan to manage any pain you might have. Many doctors apply a local anesthetic to the wound before sewing it up, to decrease the amount of pain you have immediately after surgery. If you want your advocate with you as soon as the procedure is over, let the doctor know.

Either the nurse or the anesthesia professional will start your IV. This is the time to ask for a local anesthetic to minimize the discomfort. At some point, you'll be given an IV medication to help you relax, and after that, it's smooth sailing. (These drugs have become very good in recent years.)

While You Were Out ...

As soon as you're wheeled away for your procedure, your advocate will be told where to wait. The doctor traditionally gives a report to a family member as soon as the procedure is over. Some enlightened institutions offer pagers to people in the waiting areas, so they can move around freely and not worry about missing the chance to talk to the doctor. Your advocate can use a cell phone for this same purpose. He or she can simply give the number to the volunteer or clerk in charge of the waiting room crowd and go to the cafeteria or gift shop to pass the time.

Waking Up

Waking up is a pretty disorienting experience. You may find it hard to believe that the procedure is over. If you've had surgery, you could wake up to considerable pain. Let the staff know that you're hurting; the sooner you get pain medication, the better. If you've had general anesthesia you might have a sore throat. Sometimes people wake up with nausea. Whatever your discomfort, let the staff know. They should have any medication you may need at their fingertips. If you want to see your advocate, let the staff know. They like to wait until you're pretty much awake and looking better before they let anyone in.

Traveler's Tales

When my husband had day surgery, the doctor came and talked to me in the waiting area and said everything was fine, and that I could see him soon. About every 10 minutes, I went up to the desk, asking to see my husband. Each time the clerk called back to recovery and then told me, "He's resting now. We'll let you in when he wakes up." When I heard this for the fifth time, I'd had enough. "If he's resting, then I'll just watch him rest, but I want to see my husband. Now!" They reluctantly let me into the recovery area, and there he was, wild-eyed and giving the staff holy hell. He calmed down almost immediately when I talked to him.

This made me so angry! I guess "resting" was their code word for "crazy wild." Who do those people think they are, deciding that I couldn't handle seeing my husband like that? Did it ever occur to them that what he needed most of all was a familiar face?

If you make sure that everyone, from the doctor to the guy who cleans the floor, knows that you expect to see your advocate immediately after your procedure, they will probably honor your request. If it's not honored, your advocate should move up the chain of command until there is a reasonable explanation for the delay.

Getting Comfortable

When you wake up from surgery, you'll probably be asked to rate your pain on a scale of 0-10, with 10 representing the worst pain you can imagine. Be perfectly honest when you rate your pain. Your response is absolutely subjective; only you can say how much you're hurting.

Traveler's Tales

I woke up from surgery in severe pain, and several doses of IV pain medication didn't help that much. I kept telling the nurses, and they gave me a couple more shots in my IV, and then a pain pill, but it just wasn't enough.

As they were wheeling me out to the car, I ran into the surgeon's assistant. She asked how I was doing, and I told her how much I was hurting. She said, "You should have asked the nurses to call me. I would have gotten you stronger medication."

It's your advocate's job to make sure you're comfortable. Whenever you're given pain medication, your advocate should ask how long it will take to work, and then watch the clock. If you're still in severe pain, your advocate should call the nurse. If what the nurses are doing just doesn't work, ask for the doctor to be called. If the nurses won't call the doctor, your advocate should call the doctor's office and ask the staff to page the doctor and pass on a message about your pain (this is why you should give your advocate the doctor's business card).

Getting Out

After the initial recovery period, you will be discharged once you've passed all the "tests" proving your body is in fairly good working order; such as going to the bathroom and drinking fluids. Your advocate should ask what the tests are! There may be a rule that you can't go home until a certain time period after your last IV pain medication. There may be a rule that you can't be discharged until your pain level is below five, so be careful about exaggerating!

On the Comeback Trail

Leaving the hospital is a glorious feeling; it's wonderful to feel free again, and the residual effects of the drugs can make you think you're in better shape than you really are. If you didn't get your pain medication filled before your surgery, ask your advocate to swing by the pharmacy on your way home. Take the pain pills as directed the minute you get them. It's much easier to control pain than to catch up with it once it's out of control.

Even if you feel like you'll be all right by yourself, it's a good idea for your advocate to stay with you for several hours, or overnight if possible.

Traveler's Tales

Here's what I remember about my oral surgery.
I was talking to the doctor about the weather as he

injected medication into my IV, and I was wearing a hospital gown. It seemed like a moment later I was sitting in the waiting room, fully dressed (including my parka), staring at my gloves and wondering how they got on my hands. Then there's a hazy memory of being in my friend's pick-up truck. I woke up with a jolt, standing in line at a grocery store with a half-gallon of ice cream under my arm. The clerk said, "Looks like someone's been to the dentist!" Then I was in my own bathroom, looking at a scary guy in the mirror with a swollen face and dried blood on his lips. Sometime the next day I woke up in my own bed, and I felt like myself again. It was the weirdest experience. I might have been walking and talking, but I was on another planet.

The nurse will tell you not to drive a car or make important decisions for at least 24 hours after discharge. There's a very good reason for this! It takes a while for the drugs to wear off, and until they do, you just can't be trusted. Even if you don't change your Will or decide to drive to Canada, you could still go wild on the home shopping network or phone friends and acquaintances to tell them things they really don't want to hear (another good reason for your advocate to stay with you).

Tying Up Loose Ends

You may have a follow-up appointment with the doctor to check on your recovery. Even if you got the "all clear" the day of your procedure, you need to make one more contact with the doctor. Call and ask the office staff to mail you a copy of the operative or procedure report, and keep it with your personal medical history for future reference.

CHAPTER 7

Bed and Breakfast
The Inpatient Experience

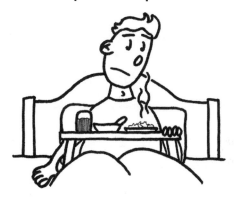

WHAT TO BRING

Your hospital room will be a temporary home, with limited space and no guarantee that your belongings will be safe. The trick is to bring essentials for your comfort, but nothing you couldn't bear to lose. For starters, you will want:

- soft cotton pajamas or nightgown, a robe and warm socks,
- drawstring pants (for times when you must wear a patient gown),
- non-skid slippers,
- two or three pillows with colored pillow cases (so they won't get mixed up with the hospital whites),
- toiletries/hair dryer,
- amusements (C.D. player with headphones, books, magazines, etc.),
- bag or sack for your personal laundry,
- cell phone or calling card to make long distance calls,
- hard candies or mints, and
- bedside journal for recording important information.

Your list of essentials should include anything that will help you feel like yourself and demonstrates your personal style. Think in terms of the five senses.

- smell: aftershave, cologne, body wash
- touch: lotion, a favorite shirt, pillow or blanket
- taste: mints, hard candy or mouthwash
- hearing: music or audio books
- sight: photographs

CHECKING IN
Request a direct admission.
Doctors are able to bypass the usual admissions process and send you directly to a room. You should ask for a direct admission if you are feeling so weak or ill that waiting in the registration area would be a hardship for you.

Ask for a private room.
This is no time to make new friends. If there are no private rooms available, your advocate's first priority should be to get you on a waiting list for one. The longer you're likely to stay in the hospital, the more important it is to have privacy. If your health plan doesn't cover a private room and you find yourself with a roommate who interrupts your sleep or sense of well being, get your advocate to arrange a transfer to another semi-private room and hope for a better situation.

Read before you sign.
You have the right to read and understand all of the papers they ask you to sign. Always make sure that all health care professionals providing care to you are on your health plan. Hospitals can be pretty lax about checking on that, and many patients are shocked to get billed in full for emergency physicians, radiologists, pathologists

or anesthesiologists who aren't covered by their insurance. You might consider writing in a clause that you will not be financially responsible for charges from any health care provider who is not on your health plan.

Out of the bundle of papers they give you, fish out the one that says "Your Rights as a Patient" and slide it into the inside pocket of your bedside journal. Any time you feel uncomfortable or uncertain, you can refer to the list of patient's rights to be sure you are receiving appropriate care. (Lots of disputes can be solved with that one little piece of paper.)

Hand over your Advance Directives.

The admissions clerk is required to ask if you have any Advance Directives, but is usually only concerned with checking this off the list. You should have copies with you; ask to have them placed on your hospital chart, and keep a copy for your bedside journal.

Insist on confidentiality.

There are federal regulations that require the hospital staff to protect all personal information about you or your medical condition. You have to give permission during registration for the hospital to even acknowledge your presence there. Other people in the vicinity should not be able to overhear your conversation with the clerk. Ask the clerk to speak softly, if necessary. You can also ask to see the computer screen to verify information, instead of repeating it out loud.

Double-check your identification band.

The patient I.D. band they attach to your wrist is your first line of defense against errors. Every time someone gives you a medication, draws blood or takes you for a procedure, they're supposed to verify your identity by looking at this wrist band. Any allergies you have are also listed on the band. Make sure this information is correct. If something's not right, tell the staff at once so they can make a new, correct wristband for you.

Your Second Admission

After the registration clerk is through with you, someone will take you to your room, and a second admissions process will begin with a nurse. You'll probably be asked three or four pages worth of questions, and some of them might seem out of left field. "Where do you turn for spiritual comfort? What religious rituals are important to you? How do you prefer to learn?" These questions come from JCAHO standards. If you wonder what they do with all the information, the answer is "probably nothing." It's only a way to prove to accrediting agencies that they're designing your care specifically with your unique needs in mind. (Right!) This is your chance to make any special requests or needs known. Are you a vegetarian? Do you want to receive communion on Sunday? Would you like to request kosher meals? Let the admissions nurse know.

Before the "flogging by questions" begins, give the nurse your personally prepared medical history and fact sheet (see Appendix C, III: Medical History and Personal Information). Point out allergies, current medications, the name of your advocate, and the list of people who can have access to your medical record.

Insist on a good room orientation. How do the T.V. and call light work? How do you order meals? What is the direct phone number to your room? Are there any restrictions on visitors?

Your advocate should ask for a unit orientation. Where are the blankets and towels? Where is the ice machine and snack refrigerator? What is the outside phone number for the nurse's station? What is the Nurse Manager's name and phone number? Be sure to record important names and numbers in the bedside journal. (See Appendix C, VI: Daily Communication Record.)

Write it Down!

When you're a patient in the hospital, you need to have a certain degree of trust in those who are caring for you. Thinking about the possibility of mistakes is unpleasant at best, but there's no disputing the facts. In every hospital in this country, mistakes happen every day. Your vigilance, and the vigilance of your advocate, can dramatically decrease the chance that it will happen to you. The single most important thing you can do is keep your very own bedside journal. You'll want to record:

MEMBERS OF YOUR HEALTH CARE TEAM
Primary Physician

Everyone should be clear about who is the captain of your health care team. Preferably, this will be your primary care physician, who already knows something about you. If your P.C.P. is not involved, then the physician at the helm will probably be a specialist addressing your major problem. On the first page of your bedside journal, record this doctor's name and office number, and keep his or her business card in a safe place. Ask the doctor when you can expect a daily visit (it's best to ask about this prior to admission, if possible). Even though doctors have very busy, unpredictable schedules, he or she should be able to tell you if you can expect a visit in the morning, afternoon or evening.

Specialists and Other Consulting Professionals

In no time at all, you can collect an amazing number of doctors and other health care professionals who are involved in your care. Ask for a business card from every one of them and record the name, specialty, and content of their conversation with you. No matter what they recommend, refer them back to the captain of the team. All decisions should be made with your primary doctor's input. It's critically important for one doctor to be focusing on the big picture. Specialists tend to wear blinders when it comes to health care issues outside their area of expertise.

TESTS AND PROCEDURES

Every time your doctor mentions a test, make sure you understand the purpose, alternatives, and any special preparations required. If you consent to the test, you should know when you can expect it to be performed. Every time someone comes to draw your blood for lab work, write it down. Your doctor will be coming to visit you every day in the hospital, and your list of questions to ask during this visit should always include a request for test results and an explanation of what the results mean. Always write down what the doctor says. This is too important to trust to memory (see Appendix C, VI: Daily Communication Record).

MEDICATIONS

When you're talking to your doctor about your plan of care, ask what medications you'll be getting on a regular basis. If you have concerns about how your pain or other symptoms will be managed, ask what medications will be available. Ask the nurse for a copy of the Medication Administration Record (MAR) so you can see what you're supposed to have on a regular basis and what medications are available to you on an "as-needed" (PRN) basis. This document is generated by computer each day and is used by the nurses to make sure you get the "five rights" – the right medication at the right time in the right dose by the right route to the right patient. If it makes the staff nervous to give you a copy of the MAR (and it probably will), just do the work yourself by writing the name, purpose, dosage and scheduled times for each medication in your journal. Any time a nurse brings you a medication, notice what it looks like and check it against your list (see Appendix C, VII: Medication Records).

Traveler's Tales

Right after I got back from surgery, a nurse came into my room and announced, "It's time for your shot." I told her I didn't think I was supposed to have a shot, but she just ignored me and started thumping the bubbles out of the syringe. With all the strength I could muster, I made an impassioned plea. "I know I'm drugged up and fresh from surgery. But I'm almost positive that shot is not for me. Would you please double-check?" She wasn't too happy about it, but went along anyway. In just a few moments, she bounced back in and very cheerfully told me, "You were right! You're not supposed to get a shot." That incident really sobered me up. You've got to pay attention every minute!

Sometimes doctors call orders in over the phone, or forget to tell you about a change. Don't hesitate to ask the nurse to double-check the order. If you still don't think it's right, refuse to take it until you've spoken with your doctor. Medication errors happen all the time, but if you're vigilant, they are less likely to happen to you.

DECISIONS

Your doctor is required to get informed consent from you every time a significant procedure is recommended. Informed consent means that you've been told why the procedure is recommended, the risks, benefits and uncertainties (see Appendix C, IV: Decision Making Guides). Record your questions and the doctor's answers.

DISCHARGE PLANNING

Your most important objective is to get what you need and then to get out of the hospital as soon as possible. Ask your doctor what needs to happen before you can go home. Aside from the primary purpose of the admission, ask your doctor how he or she will know when you're ready to leave. Does your IV have to come out first? Do you have to be able to handle a certain amount of food or fluids? Do you have to be able to walk down the hall by yourself? Knowing the discharge criteria will help you set goals for yourself. Walking down the hall after surgery isn't much fun, but knowing that it's your ticket out of the hospital can be a powerful motivator.

Sometimes discharge happens in a flurry. Don't hesitate to slow things down. You need to make sure that you and your advocate understand what new medications you should take at home, and any old ones that should be discontinued. You need to know what activities you can and cannot do, and for how long. You need to know what kind of help you'll need, so there's time to line it up. Will you require special equipment, home health visits or a change in diet? Any special instructions important to your recovery need to be explained and left with you in writing. Ask what most people complain about while recovering from a similar condition. For instance, they may not automatically tell you that most people have a weird clicking sound in their breast bone for a while after open heart surgery. Who needs that kind of a surprise? Make sure you know when to call the doctor. For every medical and surgical condition, there are common complications. You should know the signs of complications, who to notify and when. Write everything down! (See Appendix C, VIII: Discharge Planning Tools.)

Keeping a bedside journal may sound like a lot of effort, but we guarantee you'll be glad you did it. When you're in the hospital all the conversations, people, tests and treatments start blending together after a while. Depending on your memory is risky. You may be taking narcotics or other medications that can interfere with your ability to remember, or you may simply be overwhelmed by all that is happening to you.

OTHER SAFETY MEASURES
Insist on Hand washing

It has been estimated that one in 10 patients acquire an infection while in the hospital (www.cdc.gov/ncidod/eid/vol10no4/02-0754.htm). The Centers for Disease Control have determined the single most important thing healthcare professionals can do to prevent the spread of infection is to wash their hands before and after each patient contact. Health care professionals might be offended if you tell them to wash their hands, but it's so important, it's really worth the risk.

We recommend two methods. First, bring your own good-smelling antibacterial soap, so that washing hands in your room is a pleasure. If a staff member doesn't stop for hand washing before approaching you, try taking the blame on yourself. "I've got a weird thing about germs. Would you mind washing your hands?" If they say they washed before coming into your room, just tell them, "It would make me feel better if you do it in front of me." And then flash a big "humor me, I'm neurotic" smile. What can they say?

OTHER TIPS TO IMPROVE YOUR STAY

Living in a hospital, even for a short time, is never a pleasant experience. Don't miss an opportunity for self-indulgence.

1. Take your meal choices seriously. If you don't see anything that's appetizing, call the kitchen and ask for something else, like a fresh fruit tray.
2. See if the hospital has any pay-for-service options. You may be able to order movies, take-out from a local restaurant, or even a massage. (If someone who loves you springs for it, even better!)
3. When people say, "If there's anything I can do ..." give them something to do!
   a. Let them do your laundry. Send them home with your

pajamas and pillowcases.

b. Ask someone to bring your mail from home.

c. Forget the flowers; ask people to bring you good things to eat. Most hospitals will let you use the unit refrigerator if your food is labeled. Even if you're on a limited diet, you can enjoy good bottled water and fruit sorbets or ices.

4. Encourage people to respect your privacy.

a. If random people barge into your room without knocking, ask the nursing staff to place a "please knock" sign on your door.

b. Ask for a "do not disturb" sign for times when you don't want to be disturbed.

c. If signs are not available, ask your advocate to get your message across with a post-it note and a heavy marker.

d. Ask your advocate or spokesperson to let family members and friends know the hours or days when you'd like visits and phone calls, and when you'd rather not have them.

If you want to travel to exotic places, you'll have to suffer the inconveniences of shoddy transportation and unsanitary conditions. If you want to get excellent, high tech health care, you'll have to suffer the inconveniences of institutional living. It helps to remind yourself, "It might be a bad time, but it won't be a long time. I'm just passing through."

CHAPTER 8
The VIP Suite
ICU/Critical Care

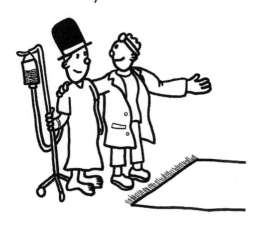

CHECKING IN

There are three ways to get into an Intensive Care/Critical Care Unit: straight from the Emergency Department; immediately after surgery (either as a planned, precautionary measure or because of complications); or from a general medical or surgical nursing unit because of a deterioration in your condition. Admission to any Critical Care Unit means that you have a real or potential life-threatening condition, so you can expect an immediate, intense blur of activity as soon as you roll through the door. The nurses have a high-speed, orchestrated way of hooking up all the monitors and alarms and setting up any special equipment, which can make you feel like you're on an assembly line. Your advocate and family members will have to wait outside at least until the nurses finish their initial work with you.

This is an incredibly fast-paced, high-tech environment. The bright lights, irritating alarms and constant parade of staff members would be stressful to a perfectly healthy person. Just the intense level of scrutiny by a nurse who is caring for you and only one other patient can be overwhelming. Fortunately, it is standard practice to medicate your pain aggressively, sedate you before any uncomfortable or frightening procedures, and provide ample doses of medication to make sure you don't care all that much about where you are. So between the medication and the illness, you probably won't have the ability or interest to be an active member of your health care team. The role of your advocate takes on extreme importance the entire time you're in a Critical Care Unit.

THE ADVOCATE'S ROLE
Priorities in the First Hours of Critical Care
Sharing important information & patient wishes

The doctors and nurses are focused on the patient at the time of admission, as they should be, but you need to make sure they have the "Medical History and Personal Information" form, the "Letter to Health Care Providers" and any Advance Directives (see Appendix C: I, Advance Directives; C: II, Letter to All Health Care Providers; and C:III, Medical History and Personal Information). Take these to the clerk at the desk and ask to have them attached to the chart. Once that information is passed on, it will take a bit of time (maybe as much as an hour) before you can see the patient. You can spend that hour notifying family members and friends of the situation, orienting yourself to the unit rules, which should be posted somewhere in the waiting room, and planning for the next step.

Understanding the Situation & Setting Expectations

As soon as the admission procedures are complete, you should expect a brief update from the nurse and a chance to see the patient. Be sure to:
- Ask for an explanation of any monitor, tube or equipment that's unfamiliar to you.
- Ask for the name and specialty of the doctor who is in

charge of the patient's care and find out when you'll be able to speak to him or her.

- Let the nurse know that you are the advocate and that you expect to be kept informed of any change in the patient's condition.
- Remind the nurse that you've left papers with the clerk to be placed on the chart. Verbally pass on crucial information such as allergies or medications that should not be stopped abruptly.
- Discuss the unit's visiting schedule. Ask if there are handouts explaining policies and procedures to the family.
- Ask the nurse to put your contact numbers on the front of the chart. (This is very important. You will need to be instantly available if consent is required for a procedure and you have been named as the health care proxy or decision maker.)

The first time you speak with the doctor, ask:

- What is wrong with the patient?
- What is still unknown about the patient's condition?
- What is the treatment plan?
- What tests or procedures are planned?
- What other specialists will be involved in the patient's care?
- How will the patient be kept comfortable?
- When do you expect to see an improvement?
- When can I expect a daily update from you? (morning, Noon, evening?)

It's very important to give this doctor the primary care physician's name and number and set the expectation that the P.C.P. will be informed and involved in the patient's care.

Some hospitals employ physicians who are "intensivists" to run their Critical Care Units. These doctors are specially trained in the care of critically ill patients and have demonstrated better outcomes. Getting an intensivist is a lucky break and a good sign that you're in a hospital that's dedicated to quality care. If there is no intensivist involved, you may want to ask the P.C.P. to coordinate and lead the care team.

ESTABLISHING A ROUTINE
Visiting the Patient
In order to best advocate for a patient in critical care, you must have access. Research has established how important contact with loved ones is to the well-being of a critically ill patient, and most hospitals have responded with liberalized visiting hours. You need to talk with the patient's family members and friends, and try to coordinate visits so you will be able to leave and keep your own life going.

Someone should always be available to meet with the doctor for a daily update and to talk with the nurse at shift change. These are the best opportunities to advocate, ask questions and show the health care team that you are involved in the patient's care. If you need to delegate these duties to someone else, at least part of the time, make sure you set clear expectations of what you're asking of them and how important it is to write down everything they learn.

Some families hold waiting room vigils, making sure someone is there at all times. Cellular phones make it possible to stay connected from a distance, but that requires a level of trust between you and the critical care staff.

Traveler's Tales

Even though I wanted to be with my dad constantly, it just wasn't practical. I had to shower, sleep, and go to work from time to time, but I could only do those things if I trusted the nurse to call me. So I developed a routine of meeting with the nurse right after each shift change. I'd size the nurse up, watch how she cared for my dad, and tell her my expectation to be called if there were any changes in his condition. Based on my first impressions of the nurse's style and response to me, I'd decide what to do. After a while, I got to know all the nurses, and my decisions were easier. If Bob was caring for my dad I could go home and sleep well, knowing that he really would call me at 3 a.m., if necessary. But if it was Carol, I had to stay through the whole shift for my own peace of mind.

Keeping Informed

The bedside journal should be in your hands, not at the bedside, during the patient's critical care stay. Collect business cards from every doctor you meet, and contact numbers from anyone who consults with you (case manager, dietician, chaplain, patient advocate, physical therapist, etc.).

Keep a running question list for your daily conversation with the doctor, and write down the answers. It's a good idea to keep a daily communication record (see Appendix C, VI: Traveling Papers), and to remember to record the scheduling and results of tests and diagnostic studies.

Apart from the uncertainty about the patient's condition, the most stressful part of advocating for a patient in critical care is the conflicting information you're bound to receive. Opinions are like noses; everybody has one. The respiratory therapist may tell you something that conflicts with what the nurses say. The day nurse may give you a completely different picture than you got from the night nurse. Specialists, because of their focus on one aspect of the patient's condition, may confuse you about the big picture. And it's easy for a story passed from family member to family member, gaining and losing details in the translation, to really mix things up. The daily update from the doctor in charge of the patient's care is your best source of accurate information.

Advocating for Comfort

Every time you go to the patient's bedside, ask yourself, "Is she comfortable?" Restlessness, fast breathing and grimacing are signs that the patient needs pain medication or sedatives. Don't hesitate to point this out to the nurse. If the patient is able to talk to you, ask about comfort. The staff will focus on the big stuff, and they can miss small, important items like dry mouth, chapped lips or cold feet.

Ask the staff what comfort measures you can provide during your visit. Can you give the patient ice chips, lotion to dry skin, or lip balm? Can you come at meal time and help the patient eat? Can you provide a shave, trim nails or give a gentle massage? Once you have permission, never ask again. Just do it.

No matter what the situation, you can always hold the patient's hand and offer comforting words. Even if the patient is unresponsive, assume she can hear.

Be sure to tell family members and friends that no plants or flowers are allowed into the Critical Care Unit. Think of comfort items that the patient can enjoy, and suggest that they bring those instead (or food for the family members holding vigil).

Honoring the Patient's Preferences

If the patient can't talk, you need to use your memory and imagination to make sure personal preferences are addressed. Who would the patient like to see? Anyone can walk into a Critical Care Unit and see a patient if there are no visiting restrictions. Ask yourself: would the patient want random neighbors or acquaintances to see him in this condition? If the answer is no, give the staff a list of approved visitors, and ask for a sign on the patient's door that indicates restrictions on visiting.

Every Critical Care Unit is a disorienting place. There is no distinction between night and day. Someone is constantly doing something to the patient or to the equipment. Patients who are alert must learn to cat nap, because even an hour of uninterrupted sleep is a lucky break.

If there's anything you can do to give the patient a little piece of normal life, try to make it happen. Does the patient love music? Bring favorite CD's, and ask the nurses to keep them playing to drown out all the bells and whistles. Hospital pillows are atrocious; bring a favorite pillow from home or buy a comfortable one. Can the patient eat or drink? Find out if you can bring in something the patient would enjoy.

Bring pictures from home and talk to the nurses about what makes the patient special to you. This has a double purpose. It reminds the patient of his "real" life and makes the patient "real" to the health care tribe. Every patient will receive the same technical care. But when a nurse can see the patient as a military veteran, award winning teacher or well-loved grandmother, the care is bound to be more personable.

Traveler's Tales

When my dad was in critical care, I had a routine. At the beginning of the shift, I would give the nurse some personal information about him. "This is my dad. He's a retired colonel in the U.S. Army. He's an occupational therapist. He's spent his whole life helping people. He is so important to us." Some of the nurses really responded to this. They started calling him Colonel and making comments about his life, even though he was in a coma.

Each day, before I left, I would ask for their help. "I have to go now because I have small children at home. Thank you so much for being my dad's nurse. Will you take care of him as if he were your dad?" Sometimes, my request would bring tears to the nurse's eyes.

Did it help? I think he got kinder, gentler care from some of the nurses because of my routine, and it certainly helped me. I needed them to know about this special man, and they wouldn't know, due to his comatose state, if I didn't share some details. They weren't just taking care of a body. This was my dad!

Planning Ahead

Critical care teams have a bad habit of springing big changes on the family without a lot of preparation. Any change in the level of care takes preparation on the part of the advocate and family members. You don't want to find out that the patient is moving out to a regular unit as it's happening. And you don't want to find out that the direction of care has changed to comfort measures only without some time to process the information and ask any questions you may have. In the daily update with the doctor, always try to find out what's around the next bend in the road. Knowing what has to happen before the patient moves to a regular unit, or what signs will indicate the treatment is not successful will make you a more prepared, effective advocate.

Ask to speak to a case manager or discharge planner early in the game. Building a relationship with this person will make transitions much smoother, and will increase the likelihood that you're not caught by surprise.

Moving Out

There are three ways to move out of a Critical Care Unit.

1. Transfer to a less intense level of care
2. Sudden (or not so sudden) death
3. Transfer to "Comfort Care Only"

1. Transfer to a less intense level of care

As soon as the patient's condition improves to an acceptable level, she will be moved out of critical care to a "step down" unit with close monitoring but a higher nurse-patient ratio, or to a regular medical or surgical nursing unit. For the patient, this can't come a moment too soon. The last day or two in critical care will probably be the worst. As the patient improves and becomes more aware of her surroundings, this environment becomes more and more distasteful.

Still, moving to a less intense level of care can be quite a shock. In the Critical Care Unit, the patient is under almost constant surveillance, and the nurse-to-patient ratio is probably 1 to 2. On a step-down unit, the nurse-to-patient ratio may be 1 to 3 or 1 to 4, and on a regular nursing unit, each nurse may care for five to eight patients, and you may only see a staff member every couple of hours. Many patients and family members feel a little abandoned when this happens.

Traveler's Tales

From the moment they admitted my brother-in-law to the ICU, someone from the family was in the waiting room around the clock. Then the doctor moved him to a "step down" unit, because he didn't need intensive care any more. Boy, was it ever a step down! We were used to him getting almost constant nursing attention. Suddenly, he was in a regular room with a nurse coming by now and again. He was still pretty much out of his head, so he needed someone with him constantly. But the entire family was exhausted. I wish we'd thought ahead and saved something for when he really needed us.

It's a good idea for someone to stay with the patient, even at night, during the first 24 to 48 hours after a transfer. If the patient was sick enough to need critical care, they still need close watching for a day or two after they graduate to a regular hospital unit.

2. Sudden (or not so sudden) death

This is not something we want to talk about, but it's certainly on everyone's mind. The patient is receiving such intensive care because of a potential or real life-threatening situation. Under these circumstances, the patient's condition can take a sudden, drastic decline, which is why the advocate and family members need to be readily available for decision making. It is important to remember that the doctors and critical care team can do everything right, and the patient still might not make it.

"Not so sudden" death happens every day in Critical Care Units. Too often, the critical care team denies the need to change directions until the very end, and that's a real shame (they do this because of Rule #10: Failure to Recover is an Insult to the Tribe). The patient endures probing, testing, treatment and procedures that have no chance of improving his condition, the entire patient/family unit has to endure the hostile, high tech environment, and critical care resources are basically wasted. The patient becomes a hostage to technology, everyone pretends there might be a miracle, and the patient dies an inch at a time.

As the advocate, your job is to speak for the patient. If the patient wanted heroic, life-saving measures carried out to the bitter end, then that wish should be honored. But many people would prefer some peace and dignity at the last. If you're wondering if it's time to stop aggressive, life-saving treatment, according to the patient's wishes, ask the doctor.

One of the first steps in switching directions is to initiate a "Do Not Resuscitate" (DNR) order. Research has shown that patients with chronic conditions or multiple organ failure have dismal rates of recovery following CPR and aggressive resuscitation.

If the patient has already been resuscitated once, and certainly if it's happened twice, or if the patient just isn't responding to treatment as expected, it's time to talk about realistic goals of care. This is very hard for the critical care team. Switching to "Comfort Care Only" makes them feel as if they've given up. This is the time to bring out the Living Will, if the patient has one, and talk about the patient's wishes.

The problem with initiating the directives in the Living Will is the requirement that the patient has a terminal condition. Doctors who are involved in aggressive treatment often hesitate to admit that there is no chance of recovery. They may put off these discussions because it's so uncomfortable for them. They may even tell themselves that they're continuing with treatment for the sake of the family.

That's why the Power of Attorney for Health Care, or Health Care Proxy, is such an important document. It empowers the designated advocate to make decisions about care, giving or retracting consent, regardless of the critical care team's desire to continue aggressive measures.

The advocate has an absolute duty, in accordance with the patient's wishes, to initiate discussions about realistic goals of care and the option to switch to comfort care. If you wait for the critical care team to begin the discussion, you may be waiting until it's too late.

There's an emotional difference for the family between choosing not to start life-saving measures and stopping them. For example, removing a ventilator when the patient is unlikely to be able to breathe on his own is a gut-wrenching decision, but morally and ethically, it's no different that deciding not to give consent in the first place.

Stopping treatment goes against the grain in critical care, and sometimes the critical care team is not very good at it. They have such confidence in their high tech wizardry that they may be convinced the patient will die the second it stops. Frequently, the patient lives for some time after aggressive treatment ends. Some hospitals have palliative care teams who can provide pain management and symptom control in these situations. If your hospital doesn't, ask for a hospice consult. A skilled hospice nurse can visit the patient in the hospital and work with the critical care team to develop a reasonable plan. You need skilled, professional help to make the transition smooth and comfortable for the patient, and to make sure that Advance Directives are honored.

3. Transfer to "Comfort Care Only"

When the decision has been made to stop aggressive, life-saving treatment, then the patient should be transferred out of critical care. Some hospitals have palliative care units for these situations. Hospice, or end-of-life care, can be provided in the hospital, in a hospice inpatient facility, in a nursing home or in the patient's home. After days or weeks in the critical care environment, it can be hard to imagine how the patient could move out to a regular nursing unit, and going home seems unthinkable. But comfort care is not complicated and can be provided very well in any setting with the right support.

A transfer from critical care to palliative care or hospice requires a big adjustment as the entire plan changes from cure to comfort. All of the testing and monitoring in critical care will be replaced with low-tech comfort measures and lots of hands-on support. A new team will be available to help with this transition, including specially trained nurses, social workers and chaplains.

In America we have the finest health care technology in the world, and the Critical Care Unit is a blessing when it works and a curse when it doesn't. Regardless of the outcome, the critical care experience is an emotional roller coaster, with an extremely vulnerable patient and an emotionally depleted family. It requires the highest level of advocacy. Because advocates are human, it is absolutely essential to take care of personal needs, respect our own limits, and seek help from family members, friends, and internal resources within the hospital at every opportunity.

CHAPTER 9

There's A Fly In Her Soup!

The Advocate's Guide to Speaking Out & Speaking Up

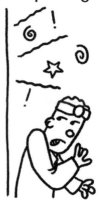

Conflict arises when a person's needs are ignored or unmet. Even the smoothest hospital stay will probably involve conflict with at least one health care professional or hospital staff member because:

1. Hospitalization is an incredibly stressful event, which makes patients and their loved ones more sensitive, clouding the ability to distinguish between wants and needs.
2. There is an unequal balance of power between the patient/family/advocate and the health care tribe.
3. The tribal rules and the principles of patient advocacy are in direct opposition, making it very easy for each side to give and take offense.

For the advocate, managing conflict in the hospital requires a three-step approach of conflict prevention, negotiation and mediation.

I. Conflict prevention

A. Building an atmosphere of trust and mutual respect

Every health care professional is an expert with an incredibly challenging job, mentally, physically and spiritually. God bless them, every one! It's important to approach them respectfully. First impressions are very important, and basic good manners are always appreciated. Be careful to never make a request that sounds like an order, or use a tone that could come across as condescending. Always introduce yourself and let the staff know that you want to partner with them for the best possible outcome.

B. Setting expectations

Health care professionals aren't used to patients bringing an advocate who will ask questions and insist on basic safety measures. Explaining why you'll be doing these things in a non-threatening way will prepare them and, hopefully, keep them from being offended. Because of their focus on the general population, notifying them of individual preferences can come across as unreasonable, so special care should be taken when you do this.

In order to make sure you don't violate the most important rules of the health care tribe (#1: The Native's Are in Control, and #2: The Natives Are Experts), it usually helps to take a "You're OK; I'm slightly less than OK" stance in your communications, which is also known as the "one down" position.

At the very beginning, when making introductions, let the staff know:

1. Your purpose and responsibilities as an advocate

"I'm Jane Johnson. You'll be seeing a lot of me, because I'm Bob's advocate. I'll be keeping track of all the tests and medications in this journal. Bob likes attention to detail, and we're afraid that, between the two of us, we might miss something important if we don't write it down. My phone number is on the chart. I want to be called if there's any change in Bob's condition, no matter what time it is. If you'll show me around the unit, I'll be glad to help Bob with little things, like ice water or an extra blanket. We know how busy you are and don't want to call on you unless it's absolutely necessary."

2. Patient Safety Measures

"If you don't mind, please wash your hands before you take his blood pressure. You're welcome to use the antibacterial soap I brought. It smells wonderful, and makes your hands feel great. I'm a little neurotic about germs. I hope you understand."

"I like to keep track of all the medication he's getting in this journal. I'll be asking what all the pills and IV's are for, until I get to know them by sight. I know you're an expert at this, but it's all new to me."

3. Individual Preferences

It's important to make these known, because even small irritations can grow into an impossible adversarial situation. At the same time, if it's not a very big deal, save your energy for things that really matter.

For example, the hospital room is the patient's temporary home, but staff can be lax about respecting that space. If some private time is required, explain the situation and ask for a "Do Not Disturb" sign to be placed on the door.

If the staff addresses the patient with condescending endearments, and it's a pet peeve, you can gently tell them that "Honey" or "Sweetie" prefers to be called Mrs. Jones. The advocate can help by referring to the patient by the preferred name, which will probably catch on.

If there are things about the hospital routine that go against the patient's grain, such as meal and bath times, you can always ask for a change. Routines are set in concrete in the hospital, so don't hold your breath that exceptions will be made unless you or the family members are willing to do some extra work to make them happen. Examples:

"Just put Mrs. Jones' dinner tray in the refrigerator when it comes at 4 p.m., and we'll help her with it around 7 p.m., when she likes to eat." Or "She's just not a morning person. I'll help with her bath in the evenings."

Communication is a weak link in the hospital, so you should be prepared to repeat the same information every time a new caregiver arrives on the scene. This can get to be tedious, but don't take short-cuts. Every single time the message should be delivered with respect, from the "one down" position.

C. Make unmet needs known immediately.

Follow the path of reasonableness, and craft your complaints in non-offensive language. Avoid blaming anyone. Simply state the issue or concern, and go for an instant resolution at the point of care.

Examples:

"He says his pain is a '10'; I can tell he's having severe pain."

Severe pain is a medical emergency, and there's a big push underway in hospitals to treat it aggressively. Most hospitals ask the patient based on new information to rate pain on a scale of 1-10, with 10 being the worst pain imaginable. The nursing staff is required to chart the pain rating before and after giving pain relievers. Thirty to 40 minutes after a pill, or 15 minutes after a shot or IV dose, the pain should be much better. If it's not, report it at once. The longer you wait, the harder it will be to relieve the pain. "Her pain is not being relieved. We want a pain management consultation."

Don't ever let them give up on controlling the patient's pain. Sometimes if the medication is not effective, the staff will find a way to blame the patient, or even you, so they can feel in control again. Pain is an entirely subjective experience, and pain tolerance varies from individual to individual. If the patient's pain is difficult to manage, a pain management specialist should be consulted.

Phrases to encourage a quick fix

"So you're telling me that ..."

If it looks like a request will be ignored, repeat back to the staff member what you're being told. For example, "You're saying that we have to wait until morning to get my sister's pain controlled?" There's something about hearing an unreasonable response or solution out loud that makes you instantly reject it, even if you're the one who came up with it.

"What does the hospital policy say about this?"

There's a hospital policy for just about everything, in order to meet the JCAHO standards. Whatever the issue, there's probably a policy that will support the resolution of the problem.

"I have some safety concerns."

Safety is a hot button in hospitals these days. If you just can't get any action out of the staff regarding an issue that's important to you, look at the situation and see if there's a safety component. If so, play the safety card, which immediately gets the natives' attention.

II. Negotiation

Negotiation involves establishing what each side really needs, and finding a way to get those needs met. Unfortunately, as a patient's advocate, the only way you can meet the natives' needs is to keep your mouth shut, which isn't likely to get the patient's needs met. When simply stating the issue doesn't result in a quick fix, we recommend that you offer a solution that would solve the problem, but would be distasteful to the natives. Your original request suddenly becomes a much better option to them. This may seem manipulative, but it's a very effective method in our experience.

This negotiation technique basically comes down to, "If you resolve this issue, I won't (fill in the blank)." To do this effectively, you need to understand what you can do that they don't want you to do. Remember the 10 rules of the health care tribe! Based on these rules, they definitely do not want you to:

- disrupt their work flow or take up their time,
- engage the chain of command, or
- aggravate their paranoia.

Negotiation Starters

"Please call her doctor."

Generally speaking, the staff would rather eat a dirt sandwich than call the doctor about a patient complaint. Using this phrase will often get you what you want, so they don't have to call the doctor.

"If you won't call the doctor, then I will."

If they try to placate you and you're still not satisfied, these words should make things happen. The only thing the staff hates more than calling a doctor for a patient complaint is having the patient, or their agent, call the doctor directly. Nothing makes them look more out of control. This phrase is just a threat, but a powerful one. If you really need to call the doctor, there's no point in discussing it with the staff. Just do it. Your doctor can verify the treatment plan the staff are following if you have doubts, make adjustments to the medications or order additional things you feel are necessary with a simple phone call to the nurse's station.

"I feel like you're not listening to me. May I speak to the hospital's patient advocate?"

Speaking to the hospital's patient advocate is a good idea. It would be nice to meet this person even before you have problems. But this phrase alone puts the staff on notice and could turn things around on a dime.

"Would you call the a) Nurse Manager, b) House Supervisor, c) Administrator for me?"
This is a tactic to enlist action. The hospital staff is dedicated to keeping complaints away from the hierarchy. If you really want or need to talk to these people, just call them yourself (see Mediation – below).

"This doesn't seem safe. I'd like to speak to the Patient Safety Officer."
This phrase escalates the action.

"I have the Medicare/Medicaid/JCAHO hotline number. Let's call them and see what they advise."
The hospital tribe only fears lawyers more than accrediting agencies. Complaints about patient care can set off interest on the part of these agencies, and interest can lead to unannounced "visits," which are to be avoided at all costs. When accrediting agencies come sniffing around, there's no telling what they'll find. These visits can turn into full blown investigations, and the hospital tribe requires time to hide any dirty laundry. So using this phrase almost guarantees that your problem will be solved, and fast.

III. Mediation
When the hospital staff and the patient/family/advocate are in conflict, and negotiation has been unsuccessful, a third party can usually intervene and provide a solution that meets the needs of both sides.

Mediation Resources
When it comes to effective mediators, the primary care

physician is your ace in the hole. As a general rule, this doctor is focused on the needs of the patient, not the needs of the hospital. The native's fear of the doctor gives him or her a great deal of power.

Sometimes the primary care physician will bow out while the patient is in the hospital, letting the specialists run the show. If the specialists are newcomers to the care team, they don't have a personal relationship with the patient and may not be as interested in advocating for the patient's wishes and sorting out differences between the patient, family and hospital staff. The patient's care may be managed by a hospitalist in the hospital or by an intensivist in the Critical Care Unit. These doctors are hospital employees, which means they'll be dealing with competing loyalties between the patient's needs and their employer's interests.

Every patient needs one doctor who is coordinating all care, including the care directed by the various specialists. Unless he or she doesn't have privileges at the hospital, the patient, or the patient's agent, can always request that the primary care physician assumes the "captain of the team" position. This is a really good idea. A lot of things can go wrong when specialists aren't aware of what the other doctors on the case are thinking or planning. Even if there are hospitalists (doctors who only care for hospitalized patients) or intensivists (doctors who only care for patients in critical care) running the show, having the primary care physician involved is an extra safety net.

If the captain of the team (i.e. attending physician) is a stranger, turn him or her into a friend as soon as possible. This doctor or his/her partner will see the patient daily while in the hospital. Use every opportunity to forge a relationship. Let this doctor know about the patient's goals, desire for information and major concerns. Get a copy of this doctor's card and keep it handy. When you have scuffles with the staff, they usually do their best to keep the doctor out of it, even refusing to "bother" the doctor for requested changes. The doctor can always be called directly. These phone calls won't be particularly welcome, which also works in the patient's favor.

Traveler's Tales

"I'm in terrible pain, and they won't do anything about it!" That's a message no son every wants to get from his mother, especially when she's 1,000 miles away and it is 2 a.m.

I called her doctor immediately and told the answering service it was an emergency. When the doctor called me back, I ranted and raved about the lack of appropriate care my mother was getting, and the doctor promised he'd take care of it.

Later, I learned about the "two phone call" solution. My call was the first; the second was the call the doctor made to the nurse's station. "This is Dr. Jones. I just got a call from a family member about this patient's pain, and I'd rather not get any more of them. Can we resolve this issue?"

I highly recommend the "two phone call" solution, because it can make problems evaporate, just like magic.

OTHER POWERFUL ALLIES AND INTERNAL ADVOCATES
Hospital Patient Advocate

More and more hospitals are filling this position, and not a moment too soon. The hospital's patient advocate can help voice your concerns, seek alternatives that simultaneously meet treatment goals and the patient's needs, and locate resources to assist you. This person is the closest you'll get to a disinterested third party within the hospital organization.

Patient Safety Coordinator/Officer

If there truly is a safety issue, such as faulty equipment in the patient's room, or medication mix-ups, the Patient Safety Officer will be more than willing to set things right. How can a Safety Officer ignore an unsafe situation?

Social Worker

By virtue of their training and job duties, social workers are naturals at patient advocacy. Ask for the Social Work, Discharge Planning or Case Management Department to find someone to help you.

Pastoral Care

A request to see a chaplain will rarely be denied. Once you get a private moment, spill your guts and beg for help.

Internal Chain of Command

1) Charge nurse, 2) Nursing Manager, 3) Nursing Supervisor, 4) Chief Nursing Officer or Director of Nursing, 5) Hospital Administrator (Vice President or President).

Move up the chain of command, or go directly to the top if you have a sense of urgency. The staff would rather have you talk to the doctor than to a hospital administrator. Hospital administrators don't want to have disgruntled patients and families. They're very busy telling happy stories about how wonderful things are. Your complaint is an ugly reminder that those happy stories might not be true. No matter what your issue, the hospital administrator will likely wave a hand and order the staff to make the problem go away.

Contacting Internal Resources

One of the biggest differences between hospitals and prisons is telephone access. In hospitals, there are telephones everywhere. To contact any of the internal resources when you need mediation, just call the hospital operator and ask for the department or title of the person you're looking for. It's that easy. Some people will only be available from 9 a.m. to 5 p.m., but because hospitals are around-the-clock operations, there is always a supervisor and an administrator on call.

External Resources

In the patient's admission paperwork, there are hotline numbers to call for issues that can't be resolved internally. These include the state health department, the Centers for Medicare and Medicaid Services, and the JCAHO. Keep these numbers handy. You'll probably never need them, but if you do, don't hesitate to call. If the patient has a private insurance carrier, you can call them for help as well.

IV. Desperate Measures

No one wants to fight with health care providers. We want to collaborate, negotiate and mediate conflicts before they get out of control. But there are times when all of these methods fail. Some situations may require radical action, regardless of the tribal rules and risk of repercussions, such as:

- safety issues,
- comfort issues,
- neglect or indifference on the part of the staff, or
- questions about the competence of the staff.

In these situations, radical advocacy may require committing the cardinal sin against the health care tribe, which is taking control of the situation. Of the 10 rules, "The Natives Are in Control" is of prime importance. Taking control is a declaration of war, and should only be the absolute last resort of the advocate.

When you travel to a foreign country, it's smart to have emergency phrases in your back pocket. Knowing how to say, "Leave me alone," "I need a policeman," and "Fire!" in the native language will be invaluable in select situations. In the same way, you need to know emergency phrases for taking control in the hospital. We hope you'll never have to use them.

EMERGENCY PHRASES
"This is an emergency!"

You can use this phrase anytime urgent needs aren't being attended, but only then. (The natives are experts and they're in control, which means it is their job to declare emergencies, not yours.)

"We'd like to see the chart."

This phrase will snap everyone to attention. Even though the patient, or their agent, has every right to see the chart, the staff will make it incredibly difficult, setting up roadblocks and bizarre rules to frustrate your efforts. The important thing here is not to actually see the chart, but to get the message across that you're not happy and you're really serious about it.

"I'd like to speak to someone from your hospital's Risk Management/Legal Department."

This is a phrase with punch. Be very careful not to threaten legal action when you talk to this person. The fact that you asked for them relays a veiled threat. Feel free to call them directly through the hospital operator. Risk managers and lawyers want you to be very, very happy. It doesn't matter if you have grounds for a lawsuit or not. They want to keep your name off their list of possible headaches.

"We'd like to have a copy of her chart."

If you've had an unproductive chat with the folks from legal, this step is certain to set them reeling. Handing over patient records is the last thing they want to do. Laws vary from state to state, but most often the hospital has to provide a copy to the patient within a "reasonable" time frame, and you get the bill for copying charges. The very first step in seeking legal action against a hospital is to request the patient's records. Even if there's nothing incriminating in the chart, your request for a copy sets off paranoia about future legal action. And the written document may help answer your questions, or help you formulate additional ones.

"The patient is talking about just signing himself out of here."

When a patient leaves against medical advice (AMA), it's a very big deal. If the staff believes this threat is real, they'll call the doctor at once. If the patient truly believes it's in his best interest to leave, call his insurance plan before mentioning anything to the natives to make sure there won't be any financial repercussions.

"The patient wants to leave. Now."

This is a serious threat and will bring the hierarchy scrambling to the patient's room. This phrase requires careful consideration, and should be used only when the patient or their agent is really prepared to carry it out.

V. Tactics to avoid
Name dropping

If you know a Very Important Person in hospital administration, or if the patient or family members know someone in power, you should never mention it to the natives. Even though there is a rigid hierarchy within the hospital, patients are seen as a collective whole. The only differences are the levels of care they require. Anything you do to insinuate that the patient deserves special VIP treatment will backfire. Having connections always helps, but you should make that contact directly, not as a veiled threat.

Threatening to call a lawyer

These are fighting words. If you mention the word "lawyer," the health care tribe will move into full blown paranoia and mount a defensive posture against you. We strongly recommend that if you feel the need to call a lawyer, don't ever say it out loud while you're in the hospital. If you need to make that call, just do it. An empty threat about legal action almost guarantees that you, or even worse, the patient, will be punished.

Displays of emotion

The health care tribe cannot endure emotional expression, especially if it's loud and in public. A public fit will get you immediate attention, but it's not the kind you want. There's nearly a 100 percent chance that you'll be labeled as mentally unstable, insane or dangerous, depending on the intensity of your outburst. If you're loud and frightening enough, they'll call security and have you escorted from the premises or even arrested.

In this chapter, we've provided ideas and examples for getting the patient's needs met in the hospital. The methods chosen in real life will depend on the wishes of the patient, the personality of the advocate, and the situation at hand. Understanding conflict prevention techniques, the negotiation and mediation resources available to you and how they interact with the tribal rules can make you an incredibly effective advocate.

The Ins and Outs

Facts About the Hospital

DAILY LIFE
Business Hours

The "powers that be" – administrators, department heads and managers, and others on the business side of hospital operations – work from 9 a.m. to 5 p.m. The atmosphere of the entire hospital changes considerably after they leave. Starting at 5:01 p.m., you'll probably notice a much more relaxed attitude among the natives.

Society and Conduct

The expected behavior of all guests, patients and visitors alike is calm, patient waiting. Very little allowance is made for demonstrative shows of emotion. If your culture or individual constitution leans toward the dramatic, don't be surprised if your normal expressiveness results in a hastily arranged meeting with the security staff.

Food

The quality of hospital food and the overall dining experience varies considerably from one hospital to the next. Some are putting a lot of effort into providing tasty, healthy meals for patients and visitors. The really progressive hospitals are adopting a room service model of patient food delivery. This may be available for family and friends as well.

If the cafeteria is closed or the food doesn't inspire you, vending machines are always available, or you can order in. Local food delivery personnel will be very familiar with hospital deliveries. Just arrange to meet them in an easy-to-find location near an entrance.

Accommodations

You could probably live in a hospital waiting room for quite some time before anyone would toss you out. Some hospitals have guest rooms for a good price, or they might have arranged deals with local hotels. More and more hospital rooms are equipped with sleep chairs or cots so that a friend or family member can spend the night with the patient.

Gathering Places

There are always lots of waiting areas in hospitals. Some are spacious and others are cozy, tucked away in little-known nooks. Families can stake out territory and pretty much claim it as their own. Often families will come to know each other, sharing space, resources and insider's tips. This is most common in ICU/critical care waiting areas.

The front lobby is usually well-decorated with fairly comfortable furniture that no one seems to use. Feel free to make yourself at home there, especially if you enjoy people watching.

You may find the hospital cafeteria to be a pleasant place to while away some time, but it's just as likely to give you a flashback to your elementary school lunch room. Nearly all have limited hours. Many visitors pass the time eating, and you can run through a considerable amount of cash between the cafeteria and the vending machines. Most hospitals have an ATM machine somewhere in the building.

Shopping

Hospital gift shops can be very pleasant to browse through. Some are incredibly well stocked, and may carry items that will surprise and delight you. These shops are usually managed by volunteers, so service and attention will vary as much as the merchandise.

Entertainment

TVs are standard equipment in hospital waiting areas, but they're usually turned on and left unattended. You can negotiate with your peers for a program more to your liking. Some hospitals offer cable TV and first-run movies to patients. If not, there may be a VCR on the nursing unit for educational purposes. If the patient, advocate or family would like to see a movie instead of "I am Joe's Liver," just ask. They can only say no. You might consider bringing your own portable DVD player from home, or one you have purchased or rented. Other entertainment options are books or music via portable CD player and headphones, which you can also bring from home.

COMMUNICATION
Information Resources
Official Information

Official information can be accessed through volunteers stationed near the front lobby, or by dialing the operator from an in-house phone. You can also approach any staff member who happens by. Health care workers have a tendency not to offer information, but they are usually fairly generous with it when asked.

Informal Networks

Families who've had a loved one in the hospital for an extended period of time get a very good handle on how things work and where things are. You will recognize them by the confident way they walk around and by the real estate they've claimed. If their children are playing on the floor with toys, if they are paying bills, or if there's evidence that they've built a virtual campground, chances are they're seasoned hospital tourists. Feel free to ask them questions. Usually they're happy to help newcomers. If you're going to be around the hospital for more than a day, it's worth buddying up to these veterans. Don't underestimate the value of this informal network.

Linking up with the outside world

It's been pretty well scientifically proven that cell phones don't interfere with medical equipment, but some hospitals still prohibit them from patient areas, especially the Emergency Department and Critical Care Units. Pay phones and in-house phones are all over the place.

Some hospitals have Internet access in public areas, and this should become more common as time goes on. You can always ask if there's an Internet portal available.

ECOLOGY AND ENVIRONMENT
Ambiance

Hospitals are like small cities. Actually, they're like small cities that were built primarily for ease of cleaning. The cold, harsh environment of a traditional hospital is purposeful. Carpet and upholstered furniture are not easy to disinfect.

Some hospitals have become enlightened about the importance of creating a healing environment. You will recognize these places immediately by the presence of living plants, water fountains and natural light, and signs that they're concerned with the comfort of guests, like basic amenities.

Climate

You can count on the temperature inside the hospital to be absolutely frigid, regardless of the season. A warm, moist environment is a breeding ground for bacteria, and hospitals don't need any help cultivating infections. Always bring a jacket or sweater.

Power

Every hospital has emergency generators to power the hospital through just about any catastrophe. This should be the least of your concerns.

Safety Codes

There are very strict safety codes that hospitals must follow or risk being shut down by the city, state or federal government. Fire safety, especially, is carefully monitored. The maintenance department is likely to be persnickety about any electrical appliances brought in from the "outside." Inpatients should declare any appliances straight away once admitted to the room. Usually the maintenance guys allow them after a thorough check.

Security Systems

Most hospitals are locked down during the night, with only one monitored entrance open from around 8 p.m. to 8 a.m., but times vary by hospital. There are usually security cameras focused on key locations in the building at all times. The tightest security in the building is around the mothers and new babies. Some hospitals have very sophisticated systems to prevent infant abduction.

Security staff can range from real off-duty policemen to barely trained rent-a-cops. We've seen these officers work very effectively in the Emergency Department, seeing that the most critically ill get appropriate attention. And we've seen others who are more than willing to escort family members from the premises for mild infractions or emotional outbursts.

Some hospitals allow their security staff to carry guns, while others just allow night sticks or heavy flashlights. A good rule of thumb: never argue with a guy who has a gun (or a bigger flashlight).

Infection Control

Hospitals are the best possible place to get an infection because of the extreme concentration of sick people. The number one line of defense in the prevention of infection is hand washing. Many hospitals provide waterless hand cleaners in strategic locations to entice the staff to wash their hands before and after each patient contact. As a patient or visitor, you will need to wash your hands often as well. You'll be touching many of the same contaminated surfaces as the staff.

Infections that are spread through the air are of greatest concern. It's a good idea to stay at arm's length from anyone in the hospital who is coughing. Hospitals are required to have negative pressure rooms that provide a separate system of air circulation so that patients with airborne contagious diseases can be isolated once they are diagnosed.

Government and Politics

Rules abound in the hospital in order to meet the standards of accrediting organizations, city, state and federal agencies, and private healthcare payors. These include:

The Joint Commission for Accreditation of Healthcare

Organizations (JCAHO) Hospitals "voluntarily" participate in the JCAHO accreditation process, but it's not really much of a choice. Refusal to participate, or failure to meet accreditation standards, results in financial disaster, because health plans will not allow their members to frequent that establishment. JCAHO accreditation is so common that failure to participate marks the hospital as a loser.

Centers for Medicare and Medicaid (CMS)

Receiving payment from Medicare or Medicaid is contingent on meeting their "Conditions of Participation," which focus on safety, quality, and most recently, patient rights. This is very good news for the consumer. Patients who are not enrolled in Medicare or Medicaid programs benefit from CMS rules, because these rules apply to all. The Emergency Medical Treatment and Active Labor Act, or EMTALA, prohibits hospitals who receive Medicare payment from refusing to treat a patient because of inability to pay without first determining that the patient is not in imminent danger. To comply with the law, an Emergency Department doctor must complete a brief physical assessment before the clerk can even inquire about insurance coverage or ability to pay. This law also prohibits hospitals from refusing to accept patients transferring from another hospital because of inability to pay.

State Health Department

Each state has a responsibility to safeguard the public from sub-standard health care. CMS and JCAHO require hospitals to post or distribute instructions for filing a complaint against the hospital with the state agency.

Federal Regulations

A federal law with significant implications for consumers is the Health Insurance Portability Act (HIPPAA), which includes privacy standards that protect patients' medical records and other health information. These privacy standards, effective in 2003, not only prohibit the sharing or release of medical records without the patient's permission, but also provide for patient access to their own medical records and protect the confidentiality of patients in public areas.

These new privacy standards have required an overhaul of hospital policies and processes regarding the sharing of confidential medical information. This affects sign-in sheets in reception areas, conversations with the patient about health or finances where others can overhear, and patient information on grease boards in patient care areas. Now, the only staff members allowed to read the patient's chart are those directly involved in the patient's care. (Which means that your next-door neighbor who works in the hospital accounting department can't nose around in your records anymore!)

Hospital Policies and Procedures

Every hospital has reams of policies and written procedures for carrying out those policies. This is basically a defensive move. By having these documents, the hospital can "prove" to regulating and accrediting agencies, not to mention plaintiff attorneys, that their standard is to always to do the right thing. If the right thing isn't done, it's the fault of individual employees, not the hospital. The problem with all these policies is that no one reads them. The good news is that they exist, and patient advocates can refer to them when negotiating conflicts with the staff.

Hospital Politics

Hospital administrative staff spends a great deal of time and effort on public relations, physician pacification and damage control. They are out of the loop as far as the actual delivery of care, but they can and will intervene on the patient's behalf for even the smallest issue if it comes to their attention.

SPECIAL NEEDS
Children

When you bring children to the hospital, it is smart to bring their favorite amusements along with you. Some hospitals have toys, books and activities for children in waiting areas, but you can't count on it. Pediatric hospitals and special children's units in regular hospitals are much better prepared for children, but it's still a good idea to bring familiar toys, healthy drinks and snacks. Waiting, the official hospital pastime, is no fun, but waiting with a bored, cranky child is pure misery.

Religious/Cultural Needs

The hospital is required to make accommodations for the religious and cultural needs of the patient. The initial assessment by the nurse will include questions about special requests, but don't be surprised if the same conversation is necessary at various points in the hospitalization. Just be patient, keep telling the same story, and insist on what is needed. You can also ask to speak to the person responsible for "diversity," translation services or pastoral care, and you can ask for help mediating with less informed staff.

Language

Every patient has the right to receive information and communicate in their native language. Many hospitals have professional medical interpreters on staff for this purpose. All are required by law to at least have translation telephones available. Even though it works in a pinch, asking a hospital employee from housekeeping or the kitchen to interpret because they happen to speak a specific language is not ideal.

Even if your native language is English, hospital staff are required to provide information that you are able to understand. Don't hesitate to interrupt "Medicaleze" to ask for an explanation in plain English.

Special Physical Requirements

Staff should be notified of any disabilities or special needs as soon as possible. Regulating and accrediting agencies require the hospital to make accommodations for visitors as well as patients.

DANGERS AND ANNOYANCES
The Calendar

New graduates from nursing schools appear in the hospital in January and June. In teaching hospitals, doctors' internship and residency rotations end and begin in July, which makes that a month to avoid if at all possible. The resident doctors will either be short-timers who are distracted by their impending departure, or brand spanking new practitioners, high on enthusiasm and low on experience. If you suspect that a doctor or nurse is fresh out of school, there are two phrases you may need to employ. "Have you ever done this before?" and "I prefer to have the Attending Physician (or Charge Nurse) do this." They need to learn on somebody, but not necessarily on you.

The Hospital Grapevine

If you have a tussle with a member of the health care tribe, chances are it will be passed on at the end of shift report. The next batch of natives will be wary of you, so it's important to turn on the charm for each new shift to dispel any gossip that you are "difficult."

Laundry

Patients should expect rough sheets from abrasive detergents (an infection control and cost-cutting strategy). It's a good idea to bring pillows and pillow cases from home. You can try bringing your own sheets, but if you're allowed to use them, don't have great hopes for bringing them home with you. They'll probably get mixed up with the rest of the laundry and you'll never see them again.

Parking

Parking is a problem at most hospitals. Some offer valet parking, which can be pricey or free, depending on the hospital's philosophy towards guests. If there is a charge for parking, it can add up in a hurry if the patient is in the hospital for more than a day or two. Stop by administration and ask if any discount parking cards are available.

Hospital parking lots can be dangerous places. If you are coming or going after dark, and especially in the middle of the night, you can pull up to the Emergency Department in your car, or stop by on your way out, and ask for a security escort. Better safe than sorry.

Who Are These People?

Making Sense of Alphabet Soup

Even if you make a practice of reading the name tags of people you're talking to in the hospital, sorting out all the initials can be a challenge. When in doubt, just ask.

MEDICAL STAFF

M.D./D.O.: Physicians can be trained through two different programs. Traditional training results in an M.D., while osteopathic training, with emphasis on a holistic, mind/body approach, results in a D.O. All doctors must pass the same state board and specialty board exams.

Fellow: A doctor who has completed residency training and is pursuing additional training in a sub-specialty.

Resident: A doctor who has completed an internship and is pursuing additional training in a specialty area.

Intern: A doctor who has completed medical school and is assisting in the care of patients for one year in order to complete basic training.

Medical Student: A student who is completing a four-year program to become a doctor.

Physician Assistant (P.A.): A professional who has had special training and passed a certification exam in order to assist the doctor by ordering medications and tests and performing some medical procedures.

NURSING STAFF

Nurse Practitioner (N.P.): A Registered Nurse who has completed additional training and passed a certification exam in order to diagnose, order tests, plan treatments and prescribe medications for patients (privileges vary from state to state).

Registered Nurse (R.N.): Title indicates a professional nursing education and a passing grade on the state board examination. R.N.s may have two, three or four years of basic training. Any string of initials after R.N. on a name tag indicates specialized training, certifications and additional degrees.

Licensed Vocational Nurse (L.V.N.) or Licensed Practical Nurse (L.P.N.): Title indicates one year of technical training and a passing grade on the state board examination. These nurses always work under the direction of the R.N.

Certified Nurse Assistant (C.N.A): This person is a technician who has completed about six weeks of training to assist patients with personal care needs, such as eating and bathing, under the supervision of the R.N. Titles vary, so this person also may be called a nurse's aide or nurse tech.

THERAPISTS

Physical Therapist (P.T.): The physical therapist is trained to identify, prevent and correct problems with joints and muscles. A physical therapist works with patients in the hospital to recover function after a medical or surgical event, and to prevent problems associated with immobility.

Occupational Therapist (O.T.): This person is trained to help patients recover or gain skills to participate in the normal activities of daily living, and to modify the living or working environment to allow the greatest level of independence following a medical or surgical event.

Speech Therapist (S.T.): The speech therapist is trained to help patients communicate. Often they're called in to identify and improve swallowing difficulties as well.

Respiratory Therapist (R.T.): This person is trained to conduct respiratory function tests, deliver respiratory treatments, and manage artificial ventilation for patients who are unable to breathe on their own.

TECHNICIANS

Just about every therapy discipline utilizes technicians. Technicians have technical training, either through a special school or on the job. They always function under the supervision of the licensed therapist.

OTHER CLINICAL PROFESSIONALS

Social Worker: This person is trained to assess needs, identify resources and coordinate services, and provide guidance, counseling and support for the patient and family.

Dietician: This person oversees the food service department and has professional training in meeting the nutritional needs of patients. When a dietician is consulted as part of a patient's care, he or she will make recommendations to the doctor for dietary orders.

Traveling Papers

I. Advance Directives

A. Advance Directives are legal documents spelling out in advance the wishes of the patient. Every patient should have both types of Advance Directives:

1. Medical Power of Attorney (also called Health Care Proxy), naming the person who is authorized to speak on your behalf if you are unable to speak for yourself for any reason.

2. Living Will, spelling out your wishes when it comes to life-sustaining treatments should your condition become terminal.

You can download a current, state specific Medical Power of Attorney and Living Will free of charge from www.partnershipforcaring.org, or have a printed copy sent to you for a small fee by calling 1-800-989-9455.

II. Letter to All Health Care Providers

This is an incredibly important letter, because it establishes your expectations about the involvement of your advocate and primary care physician, documents the existence of your Advance Directives and grants the health care provider permission to share confidential information about you and your care with specific individuals.

Whenever you access medical care, bring two signed copies of this letter with you and ask the staff to attach a copy to your chart. Put the other copy into the hands of your advocate.

Letter to All Health Care Providers

1. My advocate, _____, has my permission for full access to confidential medical information regarding my care, including, but not limited to, participation in conversations with health care providers and access to my medical record. I want my advocate with me at all times, if possible, but particularly prior to and immediately after invasive procedures. My advocate can speak for me if I am unable to speak for myself.

2. Please attach to my chart the copy I've provided of the following Advance Directives:

 ____ Medical Power of Attorney for Health Care ____ Living Will

 These documents express my wishes, and I trust that you will honor them.

3. The following individuals also have my permission to receive confidential information regarding my care:

4. My primary care physician is:

 Name:_____

 Address:_____

 Office #:_____ Fax #:_____

 If there are any complications or changes in the plan for my care, please notify my P.C.P. immediately.

 Please mail or fax a copy of any operative/procedure/lab/diagnostic reports, consultations or discharge summaries to my P.C.P.

_____

Patient's Signature   Date

III. Medical History and Personal Information

When it comes to your health, the most important tool you can have is a copy of your medical history and personal information, easily accessible and up to date. This document contains the names of all of your doctors, the medications you take, and a chronological history of medical events and illnesses. You can add anything else you think is important for health care providers to know about you.

If you take the time to complete this form and keep it current, then you can just hand over a copy each time you access health care. This one act accomplishes a great deal.

A. It will provide an extra layer of safety, ensuring that your health care providers have critical information about you.

B. It will keep you from having to rack your brain for information when you're under considerable stress, possibly leaving out important details.

C. It will keep you from answering the same questions over and over. The health care staff can complete questionnaires directly from the document, only asking you questions that aren't answered on the form.

D. It will notify everyone involved in your care that you have an advocate and ensure that your advocate's phone number is on your chart.

E. It will save time, and your health care providers will love you for it!

My Medical History & Personal Information

Name _____ I like to be called _____

Date of Birth _____ Home Phone _____

Address _____

Allergies _____

Insurance Plan _____ Group/Plan # _____

In case of emergency call _____

Phone # _____ Relationship _____

My advocate is _____

Phone # _____ Cell Phone # _____

Current problem _____

I have had the following medical problems:

Diagnosis	Date/Year	Treatment	Current Problem?
Physician			
Diagnosis	Date/Year	Treatment	Current Problem?
Physician			
Diagnosis	Date/Year	Treatment	Current Problem?
Physician			

I have had the following surgeries:

Surgery	Date/Year	Outcome
Physician		
Surgery	Date/Year	Outcome
Physician		
Surgery	Date/Year	Outcome
Physician		

I take the following medications every day:

Medication Name	For	Dosage	Frequency
Medication Name	For	Dosage	Frequency
Medication Name	For	Dosage	Frequency

I take the following medications occasionally or as needed:

Medication Name	For	Dosage	Frequency
Medication Name	For	Dosage	Frequency
Medication Name	For	Dosage	Frequency

I take the following herbal medications or nutritional supplements:

Name	For	Dosage	Frequency
Name	For	Dosage	Frequency
Name	For	Dosage	Frequency

I have had the following complications or problems from medications/treatments/surgeries in the past:

Problem/Cause/Treatment	Physician
Problem/Cause/Treatment	Physician
Problem/Cause/Treatment	Physician
Problem/Cause/Treatment	Physician

You should also know:

_____

_____

_____

Primary Care Physician Name
_____

Address
_____

Office #   Fax #

I ask every health care provider to honor the following requests:

1. If there are any complications or changes in the plan for my care, please notify my P.C.P. immediately.

2. Please mail or fax a copy of any operative/procedure/lab/diagnostic reports, consultations or discharge summaries to my P.C.P.

IV. Informed Consent

All doctors have an ethical responsibility to make sure you consent to all treatment, and that your consent is "informed." Their job is to make sure you understand what the treatment entails, as well as the risks, benefits and alternatives.
Nurses and other health care professionals may explain consent forms and ask for your signature, but the informed consent requirement is really the doctor's responsibility.

Studies have shown there is lots of room for improvement in the area of informed consent, and the blame can be shared between doctors and patients. The doctors, handicapped by time constraints and a familiarity with the proposed treatment, may not realize that the patient doesn't clearly understand what's being proposed. The patient, handicapped by the fear of appearing ignorant, the desire to be a "good patient," and the nearly universal anxiety brought on by health concerns, may not ask enough questions.

To help you understand your treatment options and ensure that you are truly informed before consenting, we've developed a decision-making guide for medical and surgical procedures. Asking the right questions and recording the answers will help you make the best decisions about your care. We also recommend repeating back to the doctor your understanding of what you've just been told, which is the best way to make sure your understanding is correct.

Decision-making Guide for Medical Treatment & Procedures

For each medical treatment or procedure, ask your doctor:

1. What is my diagnosis/what do you suspect?

2. What is the purpose of this treatment or procedure? What do you hope to accomplish?

3. How is the treatment or procedure performed?

4. What are the risks?

5. Are there alternatives?

6. What are the risks and benefits of each alternative?

7. What would happen if I don't have this treatment or procedure? (Worst case/best case)

8. When will we know the results?

9. Who will carry out this treatment or procedure?

10. What is the success rate of this treatment or procedure?

11. How much experience have you had with this treatment or procedure?

12. What preparations are required?

_____

13. Will this procedure or treatment be painful? If so, how will my pain be addressed?

_____

14. Will it require a recovery period? How long?

_____

15. Do you recommend that we do this right away, or can I safely wait until a more convenient time?

_____

16. Do you have any literature or Internet resources that will help me decide?

_____

17. Is there someone I can talk to who's been through this before?

_____

My Decision:

_____

_____

_____

_____

_____

_____

_____

_____

Questions for Your Visit With The Surgeon

1. Please describe the surgery you are recommending.

   _____

2. Is there more than one way to perform this surgery? Which method will you use on me? Why?

   _____

3. What will this surgery do for me? (worst case/best case)

   _____

4. How many of these surgeries have you performed?

   _____

5. What are the risks of this surgery?

   _____

6. Is there a chance I'll need a blood transfusion? If so, can I donate my own blood ahead of time?

   _____

7. What will happen to me if I don't have this surgery? (worst case/best case)

   _____

8. Where will I have this surgery? (If it's a surgery center not associated with a hospital, check to see if they have been certified by the Accreditation Association for Ambulatory Health Care (AAAHC).)

   _____

9. Who will provide my anesthesia? Are there options regarding the type of anesthesia I can have for this surgery?

   _____

10. Will there be doctors-in-training involved in my surgery? Will you stay in the O.R. throughout the entire procedure?

   _____

11. Will I have to stay in the hospital? For how long?

_____

12. How much pain can I expect immediately after surgery?

_____

13. How will you manage my pain in the hospital? After I go home?

_____

14. What can I expect during recovery?

_____

15. When will I be able to return to work or previous activities?

_____

16. Are there any long-term effects of the surgery I should know about? (numbness, tingling, altered function, etc.)

_____

17. When should I have this surgery? Is it urgent, or can I schedule it at my convenience?

_____

18. Can I take a tour of the facility before the surgery? (This is often very helpful for children, but can make adults more comfortable as well.)

_____

V. Information Sharing Prior to Surgery or Invasive Procedures

Outpatient Procedures

One of the most exciting advances in medical care is the ability to go to the hospital in the morning for a surgery or procedure, and return home the same day. Generally speaking, the less time you spend in the hospital, the better.

On the downside, it is difficult to properly share important information for "same day" medical events, because things happen in a hurry and it's hard to remember everything when you're feeling anxious. This form will help ensure that important information is recorded on your chart. You should also give the staff a copy of your "Medical History & Personal Information," "Letter to Health Care Providers," and Advance Directives.

Inpatient Procedures

The skill and confidence of the health care professionals in the hospital can make you believe that everything's under control, but there's always a risk of error when you transfer from one department to the other for surgery or invasive procedures. These are the times when critical information can slip through the cracks. Presenting staff with this information sheet during the preparation period right before the procedure or surgery is a wonderful investment in your own safety.

Information Sharing

Prior to Scheduled Surgery or Medical Procedures

I understand that I am to have the following procedure:

_____

_____

_____

_____

(Specify location/left/right if applicable) I have prepared for this procedure by following the instructions below:

No food since _____

No fluids since _____

Other _____

Medications I've taken this morning _____

Medications I've stopped taking prior to this procedure as instructed

Medications I've been told to take after the procedure

Allergy Alert _____

You should also know:

_____

_____

_____

Special Requests

Pain management: (low pain tolerance, previous problems with pain meds, etc.)

Symptom control: (prevention of nausea, constipation, etc.)

Other: (pre-op antibiotics if indicated, etc.)

VI. Daily Communication Records

These documents help the advocate, family and patient keep track of day-to-day developments, tests, communications from doctors, questions and answers.

Critical Care Daily Communication Record

Date

ICU/Critical Care Day #

Recorded by:

Physician responsible for patient's care today

Expected time of daily update

Primary physician's daily update

1. What are the goals of care today?

2. What has changed since yesterday?

3. What changes will you be watching for?

4. What is being done to ease the patient's pain or fear?

5. What is being done to prevent or treat complications?

_____

6. What is being done to provide nutrition?

_____

7. Other questions we have:

_____

_____

_____

_____
Specialists responsible for patient's care today
_____
Expected time of daily update

Questions for specialists:

_____

_____

_____

_____
Specialist
_____
Update

Questions for Therapists:

_____

_____

_____

1. What can the family do to speed recovery?

_____

2. Other:

_____

Therapist

Update

Primary nurse (each shift)

Questions for nurses:

_____

_____

_____

1. What comfort measures can the family provide?

_____

2. Other:

_____

_____

Scheduled tests/procedures

Results

Hospital Daily Communication Record

Date   Hospital Day #

Recorded by

Physician responsible for patient's care today

Expected time of daily update

Primary physician's update

1. What are the goals of care today?

2. What has changed since yesterday?

3. What changes will you be watching for?

4. What is being done to prevent or treat complications?

5. What can the patient do to speed recovery?

6. Other questions:

Specialists expected to visit today

Expected time of visit

Questions for specialists:

Specialist
_____

Update
_____

Primary nurse (each shift)
_____

Questions for nurses:

_____

_____

_____

1. What comfort measures can the family provide?

_____

2. How can the family help to speed recovery?

_____

3. Other

_____

_____

_____

Scheduled tests/procedures
_____

Results

VII. Medication Records

Keeping track of the patient's medications is an important safety measure. Recent studies have found that as many as five percent of all patients admitted to the hospital suffer harm from medication errors. Making sure the medication is truly intended for the patient, and that it's the right drug, given at the right time, in the right dose, by the right route, provides extra insurance that no errors will occur.

It's also very helpful to know what medications are available for pain and other bothersome symptoms. The nurses may not inform the patient or advocate about what pain medications the doctor has made available until the patient complains of pain or discomfort. Knowing up front that these medications have already been ordered provides peace of mind for the patient, advocate and family.

SCHEDULED MEDICATION RECORD

Medication Name	Purpose	Times Scheduled	Side Effects	Date Ordered	Date Stopped

PAIN/COMFORT MEDICATIONS AVAILABLE TO ME AS NEEDED

Medication Name	Purpose	How Often	Side Effects	Date Ordered	Date Stopped

PAIN/COMFORT MEDICATION LOG

Date	Time	Medication Name	Purpose	Effects	Side Effects

VIII. Discharge Planning Tools

Any time you go to the hospital, understanding discharge instructions is a very important step in your recovery. Unfortunately, this step is often neglected because of the health tribe's time constraints and your own enthusiasm for getting out of there. Being a responsible consumer and partner in your own health care requires a pro-active approach to your discharge plan. Take responsibility for asking questions and recording the answers. It will help you get out of the hospital as soon as possible and prevent a world of grief once you get home.

Setting Your Own Goals For Discharge

Asking some simple questions can help you get out of the hospital faster. Learning what must happen before discharge will help motivate you to do your part. Whether you are an inpatient or outpatient, knowing what you have to do before you can go home (i.e. drink fluids, go to the bathroom, acceptable level of comfort) gives you a sense of control.

PROBLEMS PREVENTED BY GOOD DISCHARGE PLANNING

Confusion About Medications

If you've been taking medications before your hospitalization, make sure you understand what you need to keep taking and what you need to stop taking. Find out what prescriptions for new medications you'll need before you leave and learn everything you can about these drugs while you're in the hospital.

Failure to Anticipate Side Effects

If you go home the same day you have surgery, you shouldn't be surprised by pain, sore throat or other symptoms associated with surgery. Ask your doctor what symptoms you're likely to have at home, and make sure you get prescriptions to manage them. If you are taking pain medication, there is almost a 100 percent chance that you'll become constipated. Ask what you can do to avoid this unnecessary misery.

Expecting Too Much From Yourself

Doctors and health care professionals often neglect to tell you what recovery involves. Make sure you understand what activities are recommended, and how to progress to your previous level of functioning. Knowing what you'll be able to do at home will help you plan for help if you need it.

Failure to Make Follow-Up Appointments

Find out when you should see the doctor again, and if it's your responsibility to make the appointment.

Outpatient Procedure/Day Surgery Discharge Plan

Especially in the outpatient situation, it will be helpful if your advocate completes the Discharge Plan form. Typically, the doctor arrives and gives a brief explanation of what happened during the procedure and what to expect as you recover. This occurs while you are still somewhat sedated, so you probably won't remember anything the doctor said.

Inpatient Discharge Plan

Even though you will be given written instructions at the time of discharge, they are likely to be hard to read, written in Medical-eze, and skimpy in providing the information you really need. Filling out your own sheet will ensure that all your questions are answered, problems are anticipated, and you can leave confident in your own care at home.

Outpatient Procedure/Day Surgery
My Discharge Plan

Results/findings from the procedure or surgery:

_____

_____

_____

Medications I have been given today:

Medication Name	Purpose	Dosage	Residual Effects
Medication Name	Purpose	Dosage	Residual Effects
Medication Name	Purpose	Dosage	Residual Effects
Medication Name	Purpose	Dosage	Residual Effects

Should I expect pain? _____

For how long? _____

Medication/Schedule

_____

_____

_____

What other symptoms should I expect?

_____

_____

_____

For how long? _____

Medication/Schedule

_____

_____

_____

What can I eat and drink today?

_____

When can I return to a normal diet?

_____

When can I shower?

_____

When can I drive?

_____

When can I return to work or normal activity?

_____

Special Instructions:

_____

_____

_____

_____

If I have questions, is there someone here for me to call?

_____

Name/Title

_____

Phone Number

I should call my doctor if I have these signs of complications:

_____

_____

_____

_____

I should call 911 in the following situations:

_____

_____

_____

_____

Inpatient Hospitalization
My Discharge Plan

What has to happen before I can go home?

_____

_____

_____

_____

How will the doctor know it is time for me to go home?

_____

Results/findings from my hospital stay:

_____

_____

Expected date/time of discharge

_____

Transportation arranged

Equipment or services I will need at home:

Type	Arranged by	Provider Phone Number
Type	Arranged by	Provider Phone Number
Type	Arranged by	Provider Phone Number
Type	Arranged by	Provider Phone Number

Follow-up Appointments:

Doctor/Other	Arranged by	When	Phone Number
Doctor/Other	Arranged by	When	Phone Number
Doctor/Other	Arranged by	When	Phone Number
Doctor/Other	Arranged by	When	Phone Number

New medications I should take at home:

Medication Name	Purpose	Dosage	How Often/When
Medication Name	Purpose	Dosage	How Often/When
Medication Name	Purpose	Dosage	How Often/When
Medication Name	Purpose	Dosage	How Often/When

Medications I should continue to take at home:

Medication Name	Purpose	Dosage	How Often/When
Medication Name	Purpose	Dosage	How Often/When
Medication Name	Purpose	Dosage	How Often/When
Medication Name	Purpose	Dosage	How Often/When

Medications I should stop taking at home:

_____

Should I expect pain or other symptoms after I go home?

_____

For how long?

_____

Medication/Schedule

_____

_____

_____

_____

What changes do I need to make to my diet?

_____

_____

_____

What changes do I need to make in my daily routine?

_____

_____

_____

When can I return to work or normal activity?

_____

Special Instructions:

_____

_____

_____

_____

_____

_____

If I have questions, is there someone here for me to call?

_____
Name/Title   Phone Number

I should call my doctor if I have these signs of complications:

_____

_____

_____

_____

DON'T GO THERE ALONE!

I should call 911 in the following situations:

_____

_____

_____

_____

Surfing for Answers

Reliable Health Information on the Internet

The Internet has made volumes of health care information available to all of us. The trouble is not only separating the treasure from the trash, but also finding information that is helpful to the consumer.

We want to share some basic tips that should help you make the best use of your time and energy.

1. Start searching on a reliable health care portal like Health on the Net or Healthfinder, which have already weeded out sites with unreliable information.
2. Focus on governmental, not-for-profit, and hospital websites.
3. Look for the official website for the medical specialty of interest to you. For every medical specialty, there is also a nursing counterpart with their own organization, and in most cases, an official website. Many of these sites have a section for consumers or patients, with great up to date information.
4. Look for the Health on the Net seal on health care websites (HONcode). This is a sign that the owners of the website have agreed to follow the Health on the Net ethical principles.
5. Remember that Internet research is a great way to educate yourself on available options, allowing you to prepare for conversations with physicians. Individual cases vary, and you should always review your research with a physician you trust.

About the Authors

Kathy Kalina, RN, has over 25 years of nursing experience in hospital and home care settings. She developed and refined her own advocacy skills as a hospice nurse. Currently, she's the director of an inpatient hospice, where she leads a team of health care professionals who are building a collaborative health care culture. Her published credits include *Midwife for Souls: Spiritual Care of the Dying*, (St. Paul Books, Boston: 1993). Kathy is a professional speaker and storyteller.

Stephen Pew, Ph.D., is a licensed health care administrator who began his career in hospitals and patient advocacy over 30 years ago. He was trained as a Psychologist and practiced as a therapist before beginning his career in hospital administration. His experience includes strategic planning, marketing, performance improvement, patient-focused care and the development of outcome measures for health care systems, including patient satisfaction. He holds a certificate in Conflict Resolution. His published credits include *For the Sake of the Children* (with Kris Kline), Prima Publications, 1991. Steve teaches health care administration at Park University in Missouri.

Diane Bourgeois, LMSW, MPA, has been a champion for individual and group access to appropriate health care services for the past decade. She has worked for hospitals and insurance plans, and has expertise in navigating health care bureaucracies. Diane is actively engaged in hospital improvement efforts. She is an accomplished educator and public speaker.

About Our Team

Over the years we've spent countless hours listening to the patients and their families talk about their needs and wishes, what they liked about the care they got in hospitals and what they wanted to be different. We spent an equal amount of time with the hospital staff, understanding their time, energy and resource constraints and how they wish things could be.

As a team, we're well versed in the current health care climate and hospital improvement efforts nationwide. Our professional work and continuous research has only reinforced our belief that the dysfunctional health care culture created the problems now ailing our hospitals.

Through these experiences and our lifelong commitment to improving health care we have come to believe that the best way to get collaborative care is to gain the assistance of a trained/informed health care advocate when you must go to the hospital.

If you would like to schedule a speaking engagement or workshop for your group, make a donation, or simply share your story, please contact us at: www.thepatientadvocate.org.

This book is available at quantity discounts for bulk purchases.
For information, please visit our website at
www.thepatientadvocate.org.